MORE 4U!

theclinics.com

This Clinics series is available online.

Here's what you get:

- Full text of EVERY issue from 2002 to NOW
- Figures, tables, drawings, references and more
- Searchable: find what you need fast

  Search [All Clinics ▼] for [_____] [GO]

- Linked to MEDLINE and Elsevier journals
- E-alerts

INDIVIDUAL SUBSCRIBERS

LOG ON TODAY. IT'S FAST AND EASY.

Click **Register** and follow instructions

You'll need an account number

Your subscriber account number is on your mailing label

```
This is your copy of:
THE CLINICS OF NORTH AMERICA
CXXX          2296532-2          2      Mar 05
J.H. DOE, MD
531 MAIN STREET
CENTER CITY, NY  10001-001
```

BOUGHT A SINGLE ISSUE? Sorry, you won't be able to access full text online. Please subscribe today to get complete content by contacting customer service at 800 645 2552 (US and Canada) or 407 345 4000 (outside US and Canada) or via email at elsols@elsevier.com.

NEW!

Now also available for INSTITUTIONS

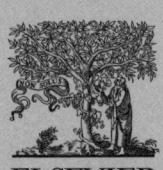
ELSEVIER

Works/Integrates with MD Consult

Available in a variety of packages: Collections containing 14, 31 or 50 Clinics titles

Or Collection upgrade for existing MD Consult customers

Call today! 877-857-1047 or e-mail: mdc.groupinfo@elsevier.com

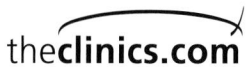

ORTHOPEDIC CLINICS OF NORTH AMERICA

Nonfusion Technology in Spinal Surgery

GUEST EDITORS
Russel C. Huang, MD
Rudolf Bertagnoli, MD

July 2005 • Volume 36 • Number 3

SAUNDERS

An Imprint of Elsevier, Inc.
PHILADELPHIA   LONDON   TORONTO   MONTREAL   SYDNEY   TOKYO

W.B. SAUNDERS COMPANY
A Division of Elsevier Inc.

Elsevier Inc., 1600 John F. Kennedy Blvd., Suite 1800, Philadelphia, PA 19103-2899.

http://www.orthopedic.theclinics.com

ORTHOPEDIC CLINICS OF NORTH AMERICA Volume 36, Number 3
July 2005 ISSN 0030-5898
Editor: Debora Dellapena ISBN 1-4160-2746-7

Copyright © 2005 by Elsevier Inc. All rights reserved. No part of this publication may be reproduced or transmitted in any form or by any means, electronic or mechanical, including photocopy, recording, or any information retrieval system, without written permission from the Publisher.

Single photocopies of single articles may be made for personal use as allowed by national copyright laws. Permission of the Publisher and payment of a fee is required for all other photocopying, including multiple or systematic copying, copying for advertising or promotional purposes, resale, and all forms of document delivery. Special rates are available for educational institutions that wish to make photocopies for non-profit educational classroom use. Permissions may be sought directly from Elsevier's Rights Department in Philadelphia, PA, USA: phone (+1) 215 239 3804, fax (+1) 215 239 3805, e-mail healthpermissions@elsevier.com. Requests may also be completed on-line via the Elsevier homepage (http://www.elsevier.com/locate/permissions). In the USA, users may clear permissions and make payments through the Copyright Clearance Center, Inc., 222 Rosewood Drive, Danvers, MA 01923, USA; phone: (978) 750-8400, fax: (978) 750-4744, and in the UK through the Copyright Licensing Agency Rapid Clearance Service (CLARCS), 90 Tottenham Court Road, London W1P 0LP, UK; phone (+44) 171 436 5931; fax: (+44) 171 436 3986. Other countries may have a local reprographic rights agency for payments.

The ideas and opinions expressed in *Orthopedic Clinics of North America* do not necessarily reflect those of the Publisher. The Publisher does not assume any responsibility for any injury and/or damage to persons or property arising out of or related to any use of the material contained in this periodical. The reader is advised to check the appropriate medical literature and the product information currently provided by the manufacturer of each drug to be administered to verify the dosage, the method and duration of administration, or contraindications. It is the responsibility of the treating physician or other health care professional, relying on independent experience and knowledge of the patient, to determine drug dosages and the best treatment for the patient. Mention of any product in this issue should not be construed as endorsement by the contributors, editors, or the Publisher of the product or manufacturers' claims.

Orthopedic Clinics of North America (ISSN 0030-5898) is published quarterly (For Post Office use only: Volume 36 issue 3 of 4) by Elsevier Inc. Corporate and editorial offices: Elsevier Inc., 1600 John F. Kennedy Blvd., Suite 1800, Philadelphia, PA 19103-2899. Accounting and circulation offices: 6277 Sea Harbor Drive, Orlando, FL 33887-4800. Periodicals postage paid at Orlando, FL 32862, and additional mailing offices. Subscription prices are $180.00 per year for (US individuals), $295.00 per year for (US institutions), $214.00 per year (Canadian individuals), $351.00 per year (Canadian institutions), $245.00 per year (international individuals), $351.00 per year (international institutions), $90.00 per year (US students), $123.00 per year (Canadian and international students). Foreign air speed delivery is included in all *Clinics* subscription prices. All prices are subject to change without notice. POSTMASTER: Send address changes to *Orthopedic Clinics of North America*, W.B. Saunders Company, Periodicals Fulfillment, Orlando, FL 32887-4800. **Customer Service: 1-800-654-2452 (US). From outside of the US, call 1-407-345-4000. E-mail: hhspcs@harcourt.com.**

Reprints. For copies of 100 or more, of articles in this publication, please contact the Commercial Reprints Department, Elsevier Inc., 360 Park Avenue South, New York, New York 10010-1710. Tel. (212) 633-3813 Fax: (212) 462-1935 e-mail: reprints@elsevier.com

Orthopedic Clinics of North America is covered in *Index Medicus, Cinahl, Excerpta Medica, and Cumulative Index to Nursing and Allied Health Literature.*

Printed in the United States of America.

NONFUSION TECHNOLOGY IN SPINAL SURGERY

GUEST EDITORS

RUSSEL C. HUANG, MD, Assistant Attending Surgeon, Hospital for Special Surgery; Assistant Professor of Orthopaedic Surgery, Weill Cornell Medical College, New York, New York

RUDOLF BERTAGNOLI, MD, Chief, Spine Center, St.-Elisabeth-Klinikum, Straubing, Germany

CONTRIBUTORS

S. AUNOBLE, MD, Département Orthopédie Pr Chauveaux, Spine Unit Pr Le Huec, CHU Pellegrin Tripode, Université Bordeaux, Bordeaux, France

HYUN W. BAE, MD, Research Director, The Spine Institute at Saint John's Health Center, Santa Monica, California

Y. BASSO, MD, Département Orthopédie Pr Chauveaux, Spine Unit Pr Le Huec, CHU Pellegrin Tripode, Université Bordeaux, Bordeaux, France

ULRICH BERLEMANN, MD, Orthopaedic Spine Surgeon, dasRückenzenstrum Thun, Thun, Switzerland

RUDOLF BERTAGNOLI, MD, Chief, Spine Center, St.-Elisabeth-Klinikum, Straubing, Germany

B. BLEY, MD, Département Orthopédie Pr Chauveaux, Spine Unit Pr Le Huec, CHU Pellegrin Tripode, Université Bordeaux, Bordeaux, France

HENRY H. BOHLMAN, MD, Professor, Department of Orthopaedic Surgery, Case Western Reserve University School of Medicine; Chief, Spine Institute, University Hospitals of Cleveland, Cleveland, Ohio

FRANK P. CAMMISA, Jr, MD, Associate Attending Surgeon, Hospital for Special Surgery; Associate Professor, Weill Cornell Medical College, New York, New York

JOHN DAVIS, MD, DDS, Assistant Professor, Department of Orthopaedic Surgery, Case Western Reserve University School of Medicine, Cleveland, Ohio

RICK B. DELAMARTER, MD, Director, The Spine Institute at Saint John's Health Center, Santa Monica, California

GILLES DUBOIS, MD, Nouvelle Clinique de l'Union, St. Jean, France

NEIL DUGGAL, MD, Assistant Professor, Department of Clinical Neurological Sciences, London Health Sciences Center, The University of Western Ontario, London, Ontario, Canada

MAHIDHAR M. DURBHAKULA, MD, Department of Orthopaedic Surgery, Case Western Reserve University, Cleveland, Ohio

PETER FRELINGHUYSEN, MD, Spine Fellow, Hospital for Special Surgery, New York, New York

T. FRIESEM, MD, University Hospital of North Tees, Nardwick, Stokton on Tees, United Kingdom

CHRISTOPHER FUREY, MD, Assistant Professor, Department of Orthopaedic Surgery, Case Western Reserve University School of Medicine, Cleveland, Ohio

GARY GHISELLI, MD, Denver Spine Center, Denver, Colorado

STEVEN S. GILL, MS, Institute of Clinical Neuroscience, Department of Neurosurgery, Frenchay Hospital, Bristol, United Kingdom

FEDERICO P. GIRARDI, MD, Assistant Attending Surgeon, Hospital for Special Surgery; Assistant Professor, Weill Cornell Medical College, New York, New York

TOMOYUKI HASHIMOTO, MD, Department of Orthopaedic Surgery, Hakodate Central General Hospital, Hakodate, Hokkaido, Japan

D. HOSTE, MD, Département Orthopédie Pr Chauveaux, Spine Unit Pr Le Huec, CHU Pellegrin Tripode, Université Bordeaux, Bordeaux, France

RUSSEL C. HUANG, MD, Assistant Attending Surgeon, Hospital for Special Surgery; Assistant Professor of Orthopaedic Surgery, Weill Cornell Medical College, New York, New York

MASAHIRO KANAYAMA, MD, Department of Orthopaedic Surgery, Hakodate Central General Hospital, Hakodate, Hokkaido, Japan

ARMIN KARG, MSc, Spine Center Straubing, St.-Elisabeth-Klinikum, Straubing, Germany

TIMOTHY R. KUKLO, MD, Department of Orthopaedic Surgery, Walter Reed Army Medical Center, Washington, DC

J. C. LE HUEC, MD, PhD, Département Orthopédie Pr Chauveaux, Spine Unit Pr Le Huec, CHU Pellegrin Tripode, Université Bordeaux, Bordeaux, France

RONALD A. LEHMAN, Jr, MD, Department of Orthopaedic Surgery, Walter Reed Army Medical Center, Washington DC

MOE R. LIM, MD, Spine Surgery Fellow, Thomas Jefferson University, Philadelphia, Pennsylvania

JOSEPH D. LIPMAN, MS, Director of Device Development, Laboratory for Biomedical Mechanics, Hospital for Special Surgery, New York, New York

H. MATHEWS, MD, Mid-Atlantic Spine Specialists, Richmond, Virginia

MANOHAR M. PANJABI, PhD, DTech, Director, Biomedical Mechanics Laboratory, Professor of Clinical Biomechanics, Department of Orthopaedics and Rehabilitation, Yale University School of Medicine, New Haven, Connecticut

GWYNEDD E. PICKETT, MD, Department of Clinical Neurological Sciences, London Health Sciences Center, The University of Western Ontario, London, Ontario, Canada

BEN B. PRADHAN MD, MSE, Research Co-Directior, The Spine Institute at Saint John's Health Center, Santa Monica, California

JOHN J. REGAN, MD, Institute for Spinal Disorders, Cedars-Sinai Medical Center, Los Angeles; Medical Director, California Spine Group, Beverly Hills, California

JEFFREY S. ROH, MD, Orthopaedic Spine Surgery Fellow, Department of Orthopaedic Surgery, Hospital for Special Surgery, New York, New York

OTHMAR SCHWARZENBACH, MD, Orthopaedic Spine Surgeon, dasRückenzenstrum Thun, Thun, Switzerland

KEIICHI SHIGENOBU, MD, Department of Orthopaedic Surgery, Hakodate Central General Hospital, Hakodate, Hokkaido, Japan

THOMAS M. STOLL, MD, Orthopaedic Spine Surgeon, Bethesda-Spital, Basel, Switzerland

ANDELLE L. TENG, MD, MS, Orthopaedic Surgery Resident, Department of Orthopaedic Surgery, Case Western Reserve University School of Medicine, Cleveland, Ohio

PATRICK TROPIANO, MD, PhD, Professor of Orthopaedic Spine Surgery, Hôpital Nord, Aix-Marseille University, Marseille, France

ALEXANDER R. VACCARO, MD, Professor of Orthopaedic Surgery, Thomas Jefferson University and the Rothman Institute, Philadelphia, Pennsylvania

SANDRA VOIGT, MSc, Spine Center Straubing, St.-Elisabeth-Klinikum, Straubing, Germany

CRISPIN C. WIGFIELD, MD, Clinical Research Registrar, Spinal Research Unit, Department of Neurosurgery, Frenchay Hospital, Bristol, United Kingdom

TIMOTHY M. WRIGHT, PhD, Senior Scientist, Laboratory for Biomedical Mechanics, Hospital for Special Surgery; Professor of Applied Biomechanics, Weill Cornell Medical College, New York, New York

JUNG U. YOO, MD, Professor and Chairman, Department of Orthopaedics and Rehabilitation, Oregon Health and Science University, Portland, Oregon

JACK ZIGLER, MD, Texas Back Institute, Plano, Texas

CONTENTS

Preface — xiii
Russel C. Huang and Rudolf Bertagnoli

Degenerative Disorders of the Lumbar and Cervical Spine — 255
Jeffrey S. Roh, Andelle L. Teng, Jung U. Yoo, John Davis, Christopher Furey, and Henry H. Bohlman

> Degenerative disorders in the spine are normal, age-related phenomena and largely asymptomatic in most cases. Conservative management of lumbar and cervical spondylosis is the mainstay of treatment, and most patients with symptomatic degenerative changes respond appropriately with nonsurgical management. Surgical intervention can be considered an appropriate and viable option when conservative measures have failed. Treatment options should always be directed toward the specific nature and location of the patient's individual pathology. Although current standards in the surgical management of lumbar and cervical degenerative disorders include discectomy, neural decompression, and instrumented spinal arthrodesis, new approaches that address this often-challenging clinical entity are on the horizon.

Advantages and Disadvantages of Nonfusion Technology in Spine Surgery — 263
Russel C. Huang, Federico P. Girardi, Moe R. Lim, and Frank P. Cammisa, Jr

> Nonfusion technology in spine surgery may improve outcomes by reducing surgical morbidity and the incidence of adjacent level degeneration; however, new technologies also introduce new short- and long-term complications. There is currently no evidence that nonfusion implants are superior to fusion in mid- to long-term follow-up. Understanding the potential risks and benefits of nonfusion technology is essential for spine surgeons and their patients. This article reviews the current evidence relating to the potential risks and benefits of nonfusion technology in spine surgery.

Biomechanics of Nonfusion Implants — 271
Russel C. Huang, Timothy M. Wright, Manohar M. Panjabi, and Joseph D. Lipman

> Although spine fusion is a versatile and effective technique in the treatment of spinal disorders, increased stresses on adjacent unfused levels lead to symptomatic adjacent level degeneration in many patients. The goal of nonfusion devices in spine surgery is to ablate or unload painful structures while preserving segmental motion. The intended performance of nonfusion devices such as disc replacement, nucleus pulposus replacement, and posterior stabilization devices can be understood from the biomechanics of the functional spinal unit in health and disease and the interplay between the motion segment and the device. Implant design issues can also markedly affect performance.

Standard and Minimally Invasive Approaches to the Spine   281
Ronald A. Lehman, Jr, Alexander R. Vaccaro, Rudolf Bertagnoli, and
Timothy R. Kuklo

> With the advent of minimally invasive surgical approaches to the spine, the ability to adequately expose the desired anatomic structures while minimizing the disadvantages of excessive soft tissue stripping, dissection, and prolonged retraction has become increasingly popular. A minimally invasive one- or two-level posterior exposure of the spine is now safely attainable with the latest minimal-access systems that exploit the biomechanics of an adjustable blade retractor. As the clinical use of these developing systems escalates, more outcomes data will become available to determine the safety and value of these minimally invasive procedures.

Lumbar Total Disc Replacement Part I: Rationale, Biomechanics, and Implant Types   293
Peter Frelinghuysen, Russel C. Huang, Federico P. Girardi, and Frank P. Cammisa, Jr

> Lumbar total disc replacement is an evolving new technology designed to preserve motion and to perhaps supplant fusion as the current "gold standard" surgical treatment for lumbar degenerative disc disease. Given the intense interest in disc replacement as a paradigm shift from fusion, this article describes the anatomy, physiology, and biomechanics of degenerative disc disease. Various treatment options and their outcomes are reviewed. A brief history of disc replacement surgery is outlined, current indications and commonly accepted contraindications for disc replacement surgery are explained, and current implants likely to be available in the United States are described. An overview of the surgical procedure is provided, with technical tips and pitfalls included. Finally, a standard postoperative regime is described.

Clinical Results of Prodisc-II Lumbar Total Disc Replacement: Report from the United States Clinical Trial   301
Rick B. Delamarter, Hyun W. Bae, and Ben B. Pradhan

> The much-awaited clinical use of lumbar artificial discs has begun in the United States. The United States Investigational Device Exemption (US IDE) clinical trial of the ProDisc-II prosthetic disc (Synthes, Paoli, PA) was recently completed, with all indications that it meets or surpasses the test of equivalence against fusion controls. This is a review of the clinical performance of the ProDisc-II artificial disc and includes an interim report from the US IDE trial at one site.

Clinical Results of Maverick Lumbar Total Disc Replacement: Two-Year Prospective Follow-up   315
J. C. Le Huec, H. Mathews, Y. Basso, S. Aunoble, D. Hoste, B. Bley, and T. Friesem

> Disc prosthesis is the new treatment for degenerative disc disease in the lumbar spine. Key to assessing the interest in this new motion technique is evaluating the results in terms of functional and radiologic outcomes. This prospective study reports the outcome of 64 Maverick devices implanted between January 2002 and November 2003. The degree of improvement was equivalent to that obtained with anterior fusion cages using the mini-invasive technique. Radiographic follow-up in this series showed a degree of mobility close to normal. The technique is safe because the intra- and postoperative complication rate is low. The Oswestry score improved for 75% of patients. This improvement is significantly correlated with facet arthrosis and muscle fatty degeneration.

Clinical Results of Charité Lumbar Total Disc Replacement 323
John J. Regan

To preserve segmental lumbar motion and to prevent adjacent segment disease, there has been a growing enthusiasm for the use of intervertebral disc prosthesis as an alternative to segmental lumbar fusion. To date, more than 100-disc prostheses have been designed, but only 10 prostheses have been approved and implanted in humans. The Charité Artificial Disc has had the longest clinical follow-up with more than 5000 implantations in over 30 countries and reported >10-year satisfactory results.

Lumbar Partial Disc Replacement 341
Rudolf Bertagnoli, Armin Karg, and Sandra Voigt

On the basis of the anatomy of the disc, the nucleus as pain generator and the resulting treatment possibilities using nucleus replacement technologies are reviewed. Various devices are presented, from the first historical steps to treatment possibilities in the future. Clinical experiences of the widely-used PDN prosthetic device are analyzed.

Cervical Total Disc Replacement, Part I: Rationale, Biomechanics, and Implant Types 349
Mahidhar M. Durbhakula and Gary Ghiselli

Cervical total disc replacement (TDR) is an attractive alternate to arthrodesis for management of disc degeneration and herniation in the cervical spine. Theoretic advantages of TDR include preservation of normal motion and biomechanics in the cervical spine and reduction of adjacent-segment degeneration. Other potential advantages include faster return to normal activity and elimination of the need for bone graft and associated donor site morbidity. This article introduces the rationale and various implant types available for cervical TDR. Part 2 of this series reviews the results and complications of specific implant designs.

Cervical Total Disc Replacement, Part Two: Clinical Results 355
Rudolf Bertagnoli, Neil Duggal, Gwynedd E. Pickett, Crispin C. Wigfield, Steven S. Gill, Armin Karg, and Sandra Voigt

This article focuses on the clinical results of three prostheses (the Bryan Cervical Disc, the Bristol Disc, and the ProDisc-C) for cervical total disc replacement. Background on the development, design, and biomechanical characteristics of each prosthesis is given and surgical indications and clinical results are summarized and analyzed.

Posterior Dynamic Stabilization Systems: DYNESYS 363
Othmar Schwarzenbach, Ulrich Berlemann, Thomas M. Stoll, and Gilles Dubois

Posterior dynamic stabilization systems have to neutralize injurious forces and restore painless function of the spine segments and protect the adjacent segments. Because degenerative disc disease has many clinical manifestations, pedicular screw systems and interspinous implants have their indications. A dynamic stabilization device has to provide stability throughout its lifetime, unless it activates or allows reparative processes with a reversal of the degenerative changes. Anchorage to the bone is crucial, at least for pedicular systems. This is a great demand on spinal implants and assumes rest and motion going together. Our experience with DYNESYS has shown that this method has limitations in elderly patients with osteoporotic bone or in patients with a severe segmental macro-instability combined with degenerative olisthesis and advanced disc degeneration. Such cases have an increased risk of failure. Only future randomized evaluations will be able to address the potential reduction of accelerated adjacent segment degeneration. The few posterior dynamic stabilization systems that have had clinical applications so far have produced clinical outcomes comparable with fusion. No severe adverse events caused by these implants have been reported. Long-term follow-up data and controlled prospective randomized studies are not available for most of the cited implants but are essential to prove the safety, efficacy, appropriateness, and economic viability of these methods.

Rationale, Biomechanics, and Surgical Indications for Graf Ligamentoplasty 373
Masahiro Kanayama, Tomoyuki Hashimoto, and Keiichi Shigenobu

Graf ligamentoplasty stabilizes the unstable segment through coaptation of bilateral facet joints. Intervertebral disc height should be preserved to avoid postoperative neuroforaminal stenosis. Biomechanically and clinically, this procedure has the potential to treat "flexion instability" but cannot correct vertebral slippage or scoliotic deformity. Surgical indication or patient selection is the key to successful ligamentoplasty. The surgical indication is degenerative lumbar disorder with less than 25% of vertebral slip, minimal disc space narrowing, and coronal facet tropism. In the long-term, Graf ligamentoplasty may reduce the risk of adjacent-segment deterioration compared with spinal fusion.

Hybrid Constructs 379
Rudolf Bertagnoli, Patrick Tropiano, Jack Zigler, Armin Karg, and Sandra Voigt

Hybrid constructs can combine motion-preserving technologies with each other or motion-preserving technologies with fusion techniques. Hybrid constructs can be implanted in single-stage or multistage surgeries. Early results are promising. Further study under formal scientific conditions is necessary to explore the benefit of these combinations.

Complications and Strategies for Revision Surgery in Total Disc Replacement 389
Rudolf Bertagnoli, Jack Zigler, Armin Karg, and Sandra Voigt

Spinal arthroplasty is an acceptable alternative to fusion in many cases of disabling degenerative disc disease. Although arthroplasty has been demonstrated to be a safe and efficacious surgical option, complications related to the approach or the device may occur in few cases. Revision strategies for failed total disc arthroplasty can be planned as a posterior fusion, leaving the total disc replacement device in place, or by way of anterior removal with subsequent anterior fusion or revision replacement of the prosthesis.

Index 397

FORTHCOMING ISSUES

October 2005
The Treatment of Unicompartmental Arthritis of the Knee
Jack M. Bert, MD, *Guest Editor*

January 2006
Oncology
Rakesh Donthineni, MD, *Guest Editor*

April 2006
The Pediatric Hip
James T. Guille, MD, *Guest Editor*

RECENT ISSUES

April 2005
Revisiting Surface Arthroplasty of the Hip
Paul E. Beaulé, MD, FRCSC, and
Michael Leunig, MD, *Guest Editors*

January 2005
Acrylic Bone Cement in the New Millenium
Dennis C. Smith, PhD, DSc, FRSCan, *Guest Editor*

October 2004
Hip and Pelvic Trauma
James A. Goulet, MD, *Guest Editor*

VISIT THESE RELATED WEB SITES

Access your subscription at:
www.theclinics.com

Preface
Nonfusion Technology in Spinal Surgery

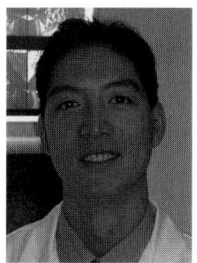 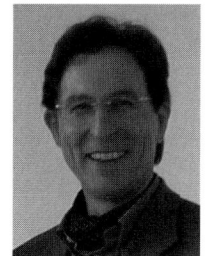

Russel C. Huang, MD Rudolf Bertagnoli, MD
Guest Editors

The technique of spine fusion was first reported independently by Hibbs and Albee in 1911. Since then, fusion has been an invaluable tool in the treatment of a wide variety of deformities, instabilities, and painful conditions of the spine. However, complications such as pseudarthrosis and adjacent level degeneration have caused spine surgeons to yearn for an alternative to fusion. Recently, efforts have been made to apply nonfusion technologies such as total disc replacement, nucleus pulposus implants, and posterior stabilization devices to a select subset of degenerative spine conditions. The articles in this issue summarize the rationale, biomechanics, and clinical results of several classes of nonfusion technologies.

Jeff Roh and colleagues from Case Western Reserve kick off the issue with a review on traditional gold standard treatments for degenerative spine problems. Russ Huang and colleagues from the Hospital for Special Surgery follow with an article summarizing the rationale, advantages, and disadvantages of nonfusion technology compared with fusion. The clinical biomechanics of nonfusion devices are then reviewed by Huang et al. A review of the standard and minimally invasive approaches to the spine follows by Ronald Lehman et al.

The next articles review the rationale and results of several classes of nonfusion implants. Peter Frelinghuysen et al, Ben Pradhan et al, J-C Le Huec et al, and John Regan review the results of three contemporary lumbar total disc replacement implants. Rudolf Bertagnoli et al contribute an article on lumbar nucleus pulposus implants. Mahi Durbhakula and Gary Ghiselli review the rationale and biomechanics of cervical total disc replacement implants. This is followed by a summary of clinical results in cervical total disc replacement by Rudolf Bertagnoli et al.

Two articles focus on posterior stabilization devices. Othmar Schwarzenbach et al describe the results of the DYNESYS implant, and Masahiro Kanayama et al report on the Graf ligamentoplasty technique.

On the cutting edge of nonfusion technology, Rudolf Bertagnoli et al then describe the use of hybrid constructs in spine surgery. Finally, Bertagnoli et al review the complications associated with nonfusion implants, and their treatment.

We hope that this issue serves as a one-stop update on the latest data available on nonfusion devices in spine surgery. Although significant data are becoming available, we also hope that the issue underscores to the reader the vast gaps that exist in our knowledge on these fledgling technologies. Widespread adoption of these techniques should not proceed until these gaps have been filled.

Acknowledgments

We would like to acknowledge the indispensable assistance of Deb Dellapena.

Russel C. Huang, MD
Hospital for Special Surgery
535 East 70th Street
New York, NY 10021, USA

Weill Cornell Medical College
New York, NY, USA
E-mail address: huangr@hss.edu

Rudolf Bertagnoli, MD
St.-Elisabeth-Klinikum
St.-Elisabeth-Str. 23
94315 Straubing, Germany
E-mail address: bertagnoli@pro-spine.com

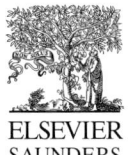

Degenerative Disorders of the Lumbar and Cervical Spine

Jeffrey S. Roh, MD[a], Andelle L. Teng, MD, MS[b], Jung U. Yoo, MD[c], John Davis, MD, DDS[b,d], Christopher Furey, MD[b], Henry H. Bohlman, MD[b,e,*]

[a]Department of Orthopaedic Surgery, Hospital for Special Surgery, 535 East 70th Street, New York, NY 10021, USA
[b]Department of Orthopaedic Surgery, University Hospitals of Cleveland, Case Western Reserve University School of Medicine, 11100 Euclid Ave, Cleveland, OH 44106, USA
[c]Department of Orthopaedics and Rehabilitation, Oregon Health and Science University, 3181 SW Sam Jackson Road, OP 31, Portland, OR 9723, USA
[d]Department of Orthopaedic Surgery, MetroHealth Medical Center, 2500 MetroHealth Drive, Cleveland, OH 44109, USA
[e]Spine Institute, University Hospitals of Cleveland, 11100 Euclid Ave, Cleveland, OH 44106, USA

The intervertebral disc is a key component in the maintenance of normal alignment and stabilization of the spine. The structure and composition of the disc support the function of the spinal segment. The intervertebral disc distributes loads and functions to promote flexibility and stability of the spine simultaneously. With normal aging, the disc becomes exposed to repetitive mechanical loads over time and eventually undergoes biochemical degeneration and dehydration. Ultimately, this process can lead to pathologic conditions.

Degenerative change in the intervertebral disc is a common and natural process in the human spine. This degeneration occurs gradually and can alter the biomechanics, stability, and neurologic function of the spine. Although these changes go largely unnoticed in most people with disc degeneration, they may manifest as back pain or neck pain and neurologic compromise in others.

* Corresponding author. Department of Orthopaedic Surgery, University Hospitals of Cleveland, Case Western Reserve University, 11100 Euclid Ave, Cleveland, OH 44106.
E-mail address: julie.bunkelman@uhhs.com (H.H. Bohlman).

The normal disc

Anatomy and composition

A thorough knowledge of vertebral and intervertebral disc anatomy is essential for understanding the pathophysiology, diagnosis, and rational treatment decisions for degenerative disc disease. A fundamental concept is the functional spinal unit, which represents the smallest segment of the spine that exhibits the biomechanical characteristics of the entire spine [1]. This segment includes two adjacent vertebrae, the intervertebral disc, and the spinal ligaments. A single motion segment is a smaller subunit that includes the paired facet joints posteriorly and the disc anteriorly. The intervertebral disc and the facet joints must support the compressive load at each level. This region has been described as a "three-joint complex" [2].

The disc itself is composed of four main components: the outer anulus fibrosus, the inner anulus fibrosus, the transition zone, and the central nucleus pulposus [3]. The outer anulus is predominantly made up of type I collagen (70%–80%) and fibrocyte/fibroblast-like cells organized in a dense concentric fashion that structurally resists tensile loads and contains the inner anulus fibrosus and nucleus pulposus [4,5]. The transition zone and the inner anulus are composed of increasing amounts of type II collagen and chondrocytes and decreasing amounts of type I collagen and fibrocytes [4,5]. The nucleus pulposus of a child primarily consists of notochordal cells; the nucleus pulposus of an adult consists mainly of type II collagen (80%), chondrocytes, and proteoglycans [1,3,4,6–10]. The inner anulus fibrosus and the nucleus pulposus have viscoelastic properties that help absorb compressive loads and help maintain disc heights [4,5]. In the outer anulus, the predominant cell type is the fibroblast [3] and the collagen fibers are parallel to other fibers within the same layer and oriented at an angle of 120° to the collagen fibers in the layer above or below [1,3,4,9]. The concentric lamellar organization is less distinct in the inner anulus. The outermost layers of the outer anulus fibrosus are attached to the vertebral body directly by way of Sharpey's fibers, whereas the inner fibers of the anulus are connected to the cartilaginous end plates that consist of hyaline cartilage covering thin cortical bone [4,6]. This composition and arrangement of the disc contributes to its ability to handle torsional, shear, and axial forces. The stability of the motion segment is further strengthened by the facets, the anterior longitudinal ligament, the posterior longitudinal ligament, the supraspinous ligament, and other ligamentous structures. A nondegenerated disc has limited vascularity and innervation to the outer anulus fibrosus.

Because of its limited peripheral vascularity, nutrients and waste products are transported by way of diffusion through this outer anulus and vertebral body vasculature [3,9,11–13]. Collagen fibers give the discs tensile strength, whereas proteoglycans help retain water and give the disc its stiffness and resistance to compression [2–4,8,13,14]. The combination of the inner anulus and the nucleus pulposus gives the disc viscoelastic properties. Logically, the discs change volumetrically when subjected to compression and bending forces, whereas changes in shape without volumetric changes occur with torque [5].

Nerve endings have been described surrounding intervertebral discs, within the anterior and posterior longitudinal ligaments, and within the outer one third of the anulus fibrosus [14–19]. Facet capsules and ligaments have also been shown to have nerve endings [4,18]. The presence of peripheral disc innervation may provide some evidence for an anatomic etiology of discogenic back pain. Two specific neural structures that are speculated to be involved in the development of back and neck pain are the dorsal root ganglia and the sinuvertebral nerves [5]. The dorsal root ganglia appears to have nociceptors for the calcitonin gene–related peptide substance P and has been found to have a high density of glutamate receptors [5,18]. The source of glutamate is speculated to arise from the catabolism of intervertebral discs. The second disc-innervating neural structure of importance is the sinuvertebral nerve that arises from the ventral root and gray rami communicantes [5]. The sinuvertebral nerve innervates the anulus fibrosus and the posterior longitudinal ligament and is also thought to be responsive to painful stimuli [5].

The degenerative process

Effects on disc composition and structure

Disc degeneration is part of the normal aging process. A key factor in intervertebral disc degeneration is a distinct alteration in its biochemical composition. In comparison to older individuals, there is a higher concentration of proteoglycans in the nucleus pulposus of younger individuals. The aggregation of proteoglycans promotes enhanced hydration that in turn accounts for the disc's resilience [5,9]. As aging progresses into the third decade, there is a decrease in the proteoglycan concentration and number of chondrocytes [3,5,7–9,13,14]. Although the mechanism for this process has not been fully elucidated, decreases in proteoglycans appear to be due to impaired synthesis and accelerated fragmentation of its structure. Loss of chondroitin sulfate glycosaminoglycan side chains leads to a proportionally higher concentration of keratan sulfate.

The amount of biomechanical loading over time appears to be responsible for changes in proteoglycans of the nucleus pulposus [20]. The net result is a decrease in the ability to maintain a hydrated nucleus, leading to alterations in disc structure and volumetric changes [3,5,7–10,13,14]. Progressing toward the periphery, the inner anulus fibrosus sustains a loss of collagen fibril organization, and the inner anulus eventually desiccates into a fibrocartilaginous material that is difficult to distinguish from the desiccated nucleus pulposus [5]. As the outer anulus fibrosus degenerates, a loss of structural organization is characterized by the appearance of cracks and fissures in the lamellae. These cracks and fissures can then coalesce into larger channels that can predispose the central disc material for herniation through the anulus [5]. Over time, the anulus becomes more histologically fibrocartilaginous and biomechanically stiff [3]. Biologically, the cells within the intervertebral disc become senescent, leading to decreased synthetic capacity and ability to replicate DNA [3].

There are several net effects on the spine that result from disc degeneration. Herniation of disc mate-

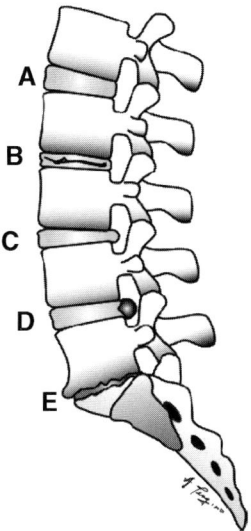

Fig. 1. Spectrum of spondylosis in the lumbar spine. (*A*) normal disc; (*B*), disc degeneration and thinning; (*C*), disc bulge; (*D*), disc herniation; (*E*), spondylosis with disc degeneration and osteophytic changes.

rial may result from anular degeneration. Depending on the location of the disc herniation, the pathologic signs and symptoms can range from myelopathy or neurogenic claudication associated with central canal stenosis to radiculopathy associated with lateral herniations. The classically described location is paramedian or posterolateral, at the insertion of the outer anulus into the vertebral body [14,21].

Symmetric extensions of the disc beyond the margins of the vertebral end plate are classified as disc bulges. The disc is considered herniated only if nuclear material is expelled through a discrete annular defect (Fig. 1). It is classified as a disc protrusion if the fragment herniates through the anulus beyond the posterior margin of the vertebral end plate. If the fragment is expelled further and the fragment is in continuity with the central disc (often by a pedicle), then it is classified as a disc extrusion [14,22]. A sequestered disc fragment has no direct contact with the disc and, by definition, migrated from its source.

Vascular and nutritional changes

With the exception of the outer anulus fibrosus, the intervertebral disc is relatively avascular. As a result, the central portion of the disc receives most of its nutrition passively by diffusion [3]. The vertebral end plates contain capillaries that support diffusion of nutrients and waste products. Studies have verified the presence of muscarinic cholinergic receptors on these end plates that may help regulate blood flow [23].

With normal aging, there is often a decrease in the peripheral blood supply; however, there are several reports that suggest that as degeneration progresses, proliferation of vessels in the end plate region adjacent to degenerated discs occurs [5]. Degenerative end plate changes can lead to sclerosis, which can further impede nutrient and waste diffusion [3]. The proliferation of vessels adjacent to degenerative discs may be the body's attempt to overcome the sclerotic barrier to diffusion in the aging end plate.

Pain generation

Pain from motion segment degeneration

Axial back or neck pain may be multifactorial and often difficult to treat. Discogenic pain, or pain originating from the intervertebral disc, is caused by derangement of the nucleus pulposus or anulus fibrosus. Degeneration of the anulus itself may lead to loss of structural integrity and eventual tearing. Painful stimuli from annular tears are thought to occur by way of stimulation of the surrounding sinuvertebral nerves.

Other possible anatomic sources of pain include the facet joints, vertebral bodies, spinal ligaments, and paraspinal musculature. Alterations in any one of these structures may adversely affect adjacent (or nonadjacent) structures of the functional spine unit, ultimately resulting in generation of pain. As the disc continues to degenerate by fragmentation and herniation, bone-on-bone apposition may result in pain with loading and motion. In addition, a collapsed disc space may lead to altered biomechanics of the functional spine unit, thereby increasing the loads on the posterior facet joints. Abnormally high loads placed on the posterior elements over time can then lead to premature facet joint arthropathy, which further perpetuates the cycle of spinal degeneration. This spectrum of degenerative changes is termed *spondylosis* (see Fig. 1). Failure of normal biomechanics or cellular structures may lead to further degeneration of the intervertebral disc [24].

Pain from neural compression

Compression of nerve roots can occur as a result of soft tissue or bony impingement. Herniation of soft disc material can generate pain by direct mechanical compression and by biochemical inflammation of neural elements. With worsening spondylosis, alterations in the biomechanics of the vertebral body and facets occur with loss in disc height. The body's response to these structural changes may result in the formation of facet joint osteophytes and osteophytes adjacent to the vertebral end plates. Although osteophytes are thought to have a stabilizing effect on the spinal segment, they can ultimately interfere with adjacent neural structures. As the disc space collapses, the neural foramen can narrow and impinge nerve roots, resulting clinically in radicular symptoms. The facets can hypertrophy and the ligamentum flavum can thicken in response to degenerative changes. With further collapse of the disc space, the ligamentum can buckle on itself and exert pressure on the dural sac. Central compression of neural elements can lead to debilitating myelopathy in the cervical spine and neurogenic claudication in the lumbar spine.

Lumbar spine degeneration

A multitude of factors such as repetitive mechanical stresses, micro- or macrotrauma, and changes in metabolism, cellular nutrition, and biochemical composition lead to alterations in the integrity of the intervertebral disc. The intervertebral discs in the lumbar spine are particularly susceptible to the process of disc degeneration (Fig. 2).

An investigation of 600 lumbar intervertebral discs found a correlation between degeneration and disc levels subjected to higher mechanical stresses [25]. Intervertebral discs in male subjects were found to have more degenerative changes than intervertebral discs in female subjects at corresponding ages. The investigators suggested that a longer avascular pathway for nutrition could contribute to this finding [25]. Degeneration of the lumbar intervertebral disc can manifest as loss of disc height, alterations in segmental biomechanics, and neural compromise.

The innervation of the lumbar intervertebral disc appears to be anatomically limited to the outer anulus fibrosus. Immunohistochemical studies have shown that nerve endings in the normal human lumbar intervertebral disc are found to penetrate only a few millimeters into the outer anulus [16,18]. With progressive degeneration, however, increased numbers of nerve fibers are found in the inner portions of the intervertebral discs [16]. These nerve fibers have been shown to be positive for immunohistochemical staining for the pain neurotransmitter known as substance P [16,18]. Inflammation and the subsequent cascade of cytokines can lead to stimulation of pain fibers in the disc and in other components of the functional spine unit [26].

Changes in the anulus can alter its structural integrity and eventually lead to herniation of the nucleus pulposus. Abnormalities in disc composition and structure, however, are common incidental findings and do not necessarily result in symptoms such as low back pain and sciatica. An MRI lumbar study of 98 asymptomatic subjects revealed that 52% of individuals had a one-level disc bulge, 27% of individuals had a disc protrusion, and 1% of individuals had a disc extrusion [22]. Similarly, other reports have suggested that positive findings on MRI do not necessarily correlate with low back pain and that degenerative changes may indeed be present in MRI scans of asymptomatic individuals [27–31].

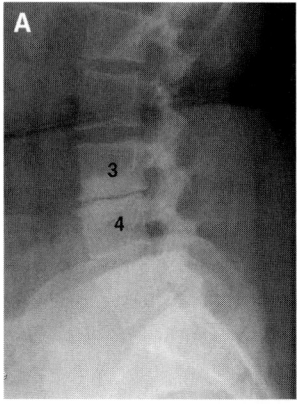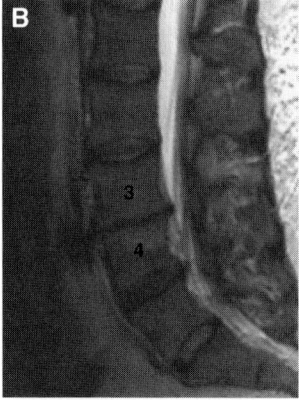

Fig. 2. Lateral radiograph (*A*) and T2-weighted MRI (*B*) of an individual with intervertebral disc space collapse, end plate sclerosis, and osteophytes between the third and fourth lumbar vertebrae.

Cervical spine degeneration

Although degeneration of the cervical spine occurs as normal age-related changes, notable differences in the anatomy and loading characteristics between cervical and lumbar spines result in differences in the pattern of involvement, rate of degeneration, and clinical presentation. Similar to its function in the lumbar spine, the intervertebral discs in the cervical spine function to provide stability, facilitate movement, absorb shock, and separate the vertebral bodies and intervertebral foramen of the cervical spine. Unlike the lumbar spine, however, the cervical intervertebral discs experience significantly less axial loads over time. Whereas the lumbar spine supports the loads produced by an individual's head, neck, arms, and trunk, the cervical spine is responsible only for supporting the load of an individual's head.

Anatomically, the cervical spine is also characterized by the presence of uncovertebral joints [32]. The joints of Luschka contain fibrocartilage that can narrow and form osteophytes during the course of degeneration (Fig. 3). Although the uncovertebral joints are less than one third of the normal disc height, they are able to bear some of the axial loads imparted to the cervical spine, thereby decreasing the overall loads placed on the intervertebral discs [33]. These factors help to make the clinical entity of cervical disc herniations rare in individuals younger than 30 years and more common later, during the fifth and sixth decades of life.

Although the presence of cervical spondylosis can manifest symptomatically as neck pain, upper extremity radiculopathy, or myelopathy, most age-related degenerative changes remain asymptomatic [34]. Similar to lumbar spine MRI studies in asymptomatic individuals, a prospective investigation of cervical spine MRI scans revealed abnormalities in 19% of asymptomatic subjects [34]. These findings suggest that MRI changes normally considered signs of cervical spondylosis (eg, degenerative discs, osteophytes, disc-space narrowing, foraminal stenosis, and cord impingement) can occur in individuals who are symptom-free. Furthermore, the prevalence of abnormalities in individuals who were older than 40 years (28%) was twice the prevalence of abnormalities in individuals less than 40 years old (14%), indicating that these abnormal changes become more prevalent with increasing age, even in asymptomatic individuals.

The clinical presentation of symptomatic cervical spondylosis is largely dependent on the anatomic location of the pathology. Cervical degeneration without nerve root or cord impingement may result in neck pain without radicular or myelopathic involvement. Anatomic studies have confirmed that the intervertebral disc in the cervical spine is innervated by the sinuvertebral nerve, a branch of the ventral nerve root [35]. Branches of the nerve innervate the outer layers of the anulus fibrosus, the posterior longitudinal ligament, the vertebral periosteum, and even the cervical pedicle.

Impingement or inflammation of the cervical nerve roots from a soft tissue or bony source usually manifests as occipital, posterior neck, shoulder, or upper-extremity radicular symptoms. Radicular manifestation of pain in a dermatomal or myotomal pattern can be provoked by direct mechanical compression or radiculitis in which proteoglycans and phospholipases from a herniated nucleus pulposus mediate a biochemical inflammation. Reproducible patterns of pain have been generated by performing cervical discography at different cervical intervertebral levels [36]. Similar studies that investigated the pain patterns produced by zygapophyseal joint injections also suggest that reproducible patterns of pain can be elicited and then blocked by selectively injecting facet joints and dorsal primary rami at different cervical levels [37–39].

Cervical myelopathy with associated lower-extremity gait disturbances, loss of upper-extremity fine motor control, and bowel/bladder dysfunction usually results from direct spinal cord compression [40]. Degenerative changes in the intervertebral disc space that can result in cord compromise most commonly occur at the C5-6 level, followed by the C6-7 and C4-5 levels (Fig. 4). Anteriorly, the cord is most often compromised by soft disc herniations, end plate osteophytes, and ossification of the posterior longitudinal ligaments. Posteriorly, cord compression typically occurs as a result of facet joint hypertrophy

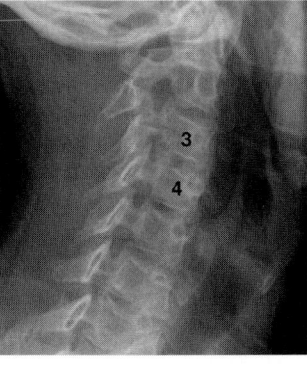

Fig. 3. Oblique cervical spine radiograph demonstrates C3-4 foraminal stenosis resulting from uncovertebral osteophyte impingement.

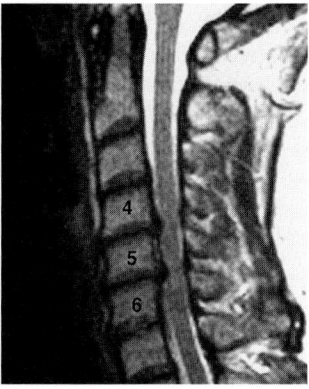

Fig. 4. Cervical T2-weighted MRI reveals herniated discs with cord impingement at C4-5 and C5-6.

and buckling of the ligamentum flavum. Perhaps the most important determinant of symptomatic manifestation of myelopathy is the space available for the spinal cord. Degenerative changes in the cervical spine can lead to an overall decrease in this space (Fig. 5). An investigation of 100 consecutive surgical patients with cervical disc herniations revealed that the spinal canal sagittal diameters and cross-sectional areas in patients with motor disturbances were significantly smaller than in asymptomatic healthy controls [41]. Progressive narrowing of the spinal canal with resultant compression of the spinal cord can eventually lead to worsening disability and deterioration of normal function [42].

Treatment of degenerative disorders

Conservative treatment remains the standard of care in the symptomatic treatment of degenerative disc disease [43]. Modalities including nonsteroidal anti-inflammatory medications, analgesics, short-term bed rest, physical therapy, heat, electrical therapy, and lifestyle modifications represent some of the mainstays in the management of lumbar and cervical spinal degeneration. Spinal injections (including epidural, selective nerve root, and facet joint injections) can serve dual diagnostic and therapeutic roles [44–47]. As diagnostic tools, selective nerve root and facet joint injections can often accurately identify the precise symptomatic level, help confirm a suspected diagnosis, and allow the clinician to design a more focused and individualized treatment approach. As therapeutic modalities, injections can provide symptomatic relief and a pain-free window to allow for more aggressive physiotherapy.

Although controversial as a diagnostic test, provocative discography is often employed as technique to identify symptomatic disc levels [48]. It is often cited as the only procedure that can determine whether a specific disc is the true generator of pain. After localization into the nucleus pulposus, contrast dye is injected to assess internal disc morphology and to provoke a pain response. Discography may be a useful diagnostic procedure in symptomatic patients who have no definitive diagnostic imaging studies or when clinical symptoms require radiologic correlation [49]. If concordant pain is elicited on discographic evaluation, the level in question may be amenable to surgical intervention.

When conservative measures fail, surgical options have traditionally included decompression of neural elements and arthrodesis of painful, diseased spinal segments or surgical excision of diseased intervertebral discs with their associated nociceptors [50]. In the lumbar spine, multiple surgical options are available in the surgeon's armamentarium, including central/foraminal decompression, posterolateral fusion, posterior lumbar interbody fusion, transforaminal lumbar interbody fusion, and anterior lumbar interbody fusion. The decision to include spinal instrumentation must be based on factors such as deformity correction and stabilization before fusion consolidation and must be made at the discretion of the operating surgeon.

In the cervical spine, anterior and posterior approaches have been successfully implemented in the treatment of degenerative disorders. The specific approach and surgical treatment must cater to the specific nature and location of each patient's own cervical pathology. Historically, however, cervical spondylotic radiculopathy and myelopathy have most commonly

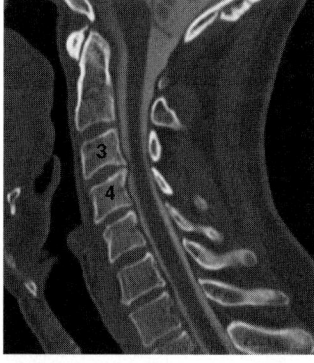

Fig. 5. Sagittal CT reconstruction of the cervical spine confirms central stenosis from end plate osteophytes with a notable decrease in the space available for the spinal cord at the C3-4 level.

been successfully treated with anterior cervical decompression and arthrodesis [51,52]. Discectomy, neural decompression, and segmental arthrodesis, with attention to careful end plate preparation, have become the mainstays in the surgical management of degenerative disc disease and spondylosis [53].

The future of degenerative disc treatment includes newly developed strategies aimed at preventing degenerative disc disease or regenerating degenerated discs [5,54]. Spinal arthroplasty (including intervertebral disc and facet joint replacement) is a novel surgical alternative with the potential benefit of relieving back and neck pain while maintaining segmental motion [50].

Summary

The etiology of symptom manifestation in lumbar and cervical spine degeneration is multifactorial and includes cellular, biochemical, and biomechanical causes. Accurate identification of pain generators in the degenerative spine can be challenging. After a diagnosis is made, however, treatment measures must address the patient's pain, neurologic function, and spinal stability. The clinician must understand that degenerative disorders in the spine are normal, age-related phenomena and largely asymptomatic in most cases. Conservative management of lumbar and cervical spondylosis is the mainstay of treatment, and most patients with symptomatic degenerative changes respond appropriately with nonsurgical management. Only when conservative measures have failed can surgical intervention be considered an appropriate and viable option. Treatment options should always be directed toward the specific nature and location of the patient's individual pathology. Although current standards in the surgical management of lumbar and cervical degenerative disorders include discectomy, neural decompression, and instrumented spinal arthrodesis, new approaches that address this often-challenging clinical entity are on the horizon.

References

[1] Yaszemski MJ, White A, Panjabi M. Biomechanics of the spine. In: Fardon DF, Garfin SR, editors. Orthopeadic knowledge update, spine. 2nd edition. Rosemont (IL): AAOS; 2002. p. 15–23.

[2] Yong-Hing K, Kirkaldy-Willis WH. The pathophysiology of degenerative disease of the lumbar spine. Orthop Clin N Am 1983;14:491–504.

[3] Buckwalter JA. Aging and degeneration of the human intervertebral disc. Spine 1995;20:1307–14.

[4] Buckwalter JA, Moe VC, Boden SD, et al. Intervertebral disk structure, composition, and mechanical function. In: Buckwalter JA, Einhorn TA, Simon SR, editors. Orthopaedic basic science. 2nd edition. Rosemont (IL): AAOS; 2000. p. 548–56.

[5] Biyani A, Andersson GB. Low back pain: pathophysiology and management. J Am Acad Orthop Surg 2004;12:106–15.

[6] Guiot BH, Fessler RG. Molecular biology of degenerative disc disease. Neurosurgery 2000;47:1034–40.

[7] Buckwalter JA, Smith KC, Kazarien LE, et al. Articular cartilage and intervertebral disc proteoglycans differ in structure: an electron microscopic study. J Orthop Res 1989;7:146–51.

[8] Buckwalter JA, Pedrini-Mille A, Pedrini V, et al. Proteoglycans of human infant intervertebral disc. Electron microscopic and biochemical studies. J Bone Joint Surg Am 1985;67:284–94.

[9] Chung SA, Khan SN, Diwan AD. The molecular basis of intervertebral disk degeneration. Orthop Clin N Am 2003;34:209–19.

[10] Pritzker KP. Aging and degeneration in the lumbar intervertebral disc. Orthop Clin N Am 1977;8:66–77.

[11] Humzah MD, Soames RW. Human intervertebral disc: structure and function. Anat Rec 1988;220:337–56.

[12] Rudert M, Tillmann B. Lymph and blood supply of the human intervertebral disc. Cadaver study of correlations to discitis. Acta Orthop Scand 1993;64:37–40.

[13] Buckwalter JA, Roughley PJ, Rosenberg LC. Age-related changes in cartilage proteoglycans: quantitative electron microscopic studies. Microsc Res Tech 1994;28:398–408.

[14] Buckwalter JA, Boden SD, Eyre DR, et al. Intervertebral disk aging, degeneration, and herniation. In: Buckwalter JA, Einhorn TA, Simon SR, editors. Orthopaedic basic science. 2nd edition. Rosemont (IL): AAOS; 2000. p. 557–66.

[15] Coppes MH, Marani E, Thomeer RT, et al. Innervation of annulus fibrosis in low back pain. Lancet 1990;336: 189–90.

[16] Coppes MH, Marani E, Thomeer RT, et al. Innervation of "painful" lumbar discs. Spine 1997;22:2342–9 [discussion: 2349–50].

[17] Groen GJ, Baljet B, Drukker J. Nerves and nerve plexuses of the human vertebral column. Am J Anat 1990;188:282–96.

[18] Palmgren T, Gronblad M, Virri J, et al. An immunohistochemical study of nerve structures in the annulus fibrosus of human normal lumbar intervertebral discs. Spine 1999;24:2075–9.

[19] Bogduk N, Tynan W, Wilson AS. The nerve supply to the human lumbar intervertebral discs. J Anat 1981; 132:39–56.

[20] Taylor TK, Melrose J, Burkhardt D, et al. Spinal biomechanics and aging are major determinants of the proteoglycan metabolism of intervertebral disc cells. Spine 2000;25:3014–20.

[21] Iencean SM. Lumbar intervertebral disc herniation following experimental intradiscal pressure increase. Acta Neurochir (Wien) 2000;142:669–76.

[22] Jensen MC, Brant-Zawadzki MN, Obuchowski N, et al. Magnetic resonance imaging of the lumbar spine in people without back pain. N Engl J Med 1994; 331:69–73.

[23] Wallace AL, Wyatt BC, McCarthy ID, et al. Humoral regulation of blood flow in the vertebral endplate. Spine 1994;19:1324–8.

[24] Adams MA, Freeman BJ, Morrison HP, et al. Mechanical initiation of intervertebral disc degeneration. Spine 2000;25:1625–36.

[25] Miller JA, Schmatz C, Schultz AB. Lumbar disc degeneration: correlation with age, sex, and spine level in 600 autopsy specimens. Spine 1988;13:173–8.

[26] Igarashi A, Kikuchi S, Konno S, et al. Inflammatory cytokines released from the facet joint tissue in degenerative lumbar spinal disorders. Spine 2004;29: 2091–5.

[27] Boden SD, Wiesel SW. Lumbar spine imaging: role in clinical decision making. J Am Acad Orthop Surg 1996;4:238–48.

[28] Boden SD, Riew KD, Yamaguchi K, et al. Orientation of the lumbar facet joints: association with degenerative disc disease. J Bone Joint Surg Am 1996;78: 403–11.

[29] Boden SD, Davis DO, Dina TS, et al. Abnormal magnetic-resonance scans of the lumbar spine in asymptomatic subjects. A prospective investigation. J Bone Joint Surg Am 1990;72:403–8.

[30] Savage RA, Whitehouse GH, Roberts N. The relationship between the magnetic resonance imaging appearance of the lumbar spine and low back pain, age and occupation in males. Eur Spine J 1997;6: 106–14.

[31] Greenberg JO, Schnell RG. Magnetic resonance imaging of the lumbar spine in asymptomatic adults. Cooperative study—American Society of Neuroimaging. J Neuroimaging 1991;1:2–7.

[32] Hayashi K, Yabuki T. Origin of the uncus and of Luschka's joint in the cervical spine. J Bone Joint Surg Am 1985;67:788–91.

[33] Hadley L. The covertebral articulation and cervical foramen encroachment. J Bone Joint Surg Am 1957; 39:910–20.

[34] Rao R. Neck pain, cervical radiculopathy, and cervical myelopathy. Pathophysiology, natural history, and clinical evaluation. J Bone Joint Surg Am 2002;84: 1872–81.

[35] Boduk N, Windsor M, Inglis A. The innervation of the cervical intervertebral disc. Spine 1998;13:2–8.

[36] Grubb SA, Kelly CK. Cervical discography: clinical implications from 12 years of experience. Spine 2000; 25:1382–9.

[37] Dwyer A, Aprill C, Bogduk N. Cervical zygapophyseal joint pain patterns I: a study in normal volunteers. Spine 1990;15:453–7.

[38] Aprill C, Dwyer A, Bogduk N. Cervical zygapophyseal joint pain patterns II: a clinical evaluation. Spine 1990;15:458–61.

[39] Bogduk N, Marsland A. The cervical zygapophyseal joints as a source of neck pain. Spine 1988;13:610–7.

[40] Heller JG. Surgical treatment of degenerative cervical disc disease. In: Fardon DF, Garfin SR, editors. Orthopeadic knowledge update, spine. 2nd edition. Rosemont (IL): AAOS; 2002. p. 299–309.

[41] Debois M, Hertz R, Berghmans D, et al. Soft cervical disc herniations. Spine 1999;24:1996–2002.

[42] Nurick S. The pathogenesis of the spinal cord disorder associated with cervical spondylosis. Brain 1972;95: 87–100.

[43] Saal JS, Saal JA, Yurth EF. Nonoperative management of herniated cervical intervertebral radiculopathy. Spine 1996;21:1877–83.

[44] Derby R, Bogduk N, Schwarzer A. Precision percutaneous blocking procedure for localizing pain. Part I: the posterior lumbar component. Pain Digest 1993;3: 89–100.

[45] Barnsley L, Lord S, Bogduk N. Comparative local anesthetic blocks in the diagnosis of cervical zygapophyseal joint pain. Pain 1993;55:99–106.

[46] Warfield CA, Biber MP, Crews DA. Epidural steroid injection as a treatment for cervical radiculitis. Clin J Pain 1998;4:201–4.

[47] Ferrante FM, Wilson SP, Iacobo C. Clinical classification as a predictor of therapeutic outcome after cervical epidural steroid injection. Spine 1993;18: 730–6.

[48] Bogduk N, Aprill C. On the nature of neck pain, discography, and cervical zygapophyseal blocks. Pain 1993;54:213–7.

[49] Guyer RD, Ohnmeiss DD. Lumbar discography: position statement from the North American Spine Society Diagnostic and Therapeutic Committee. Spine 1995;20:2048–59.

[50] Chedid KJ, Chedid MK. The "tract" of history in the treatment of lumbar degenerative disc disease. Neurosurg Focus 2004;16:E7.

[51] Bohlman HH, Emery SE, Goodfellow DB, et al. Robinson anterior cervical discetomy and arthrodesis for cervical radiculopathy: long term follow-up of one hundred and twenty-two patients. J Bone Joint Surg Am 1993;75:1298–307.

[52] Emery SE, Bohlman HH, Bolesta MJ, et al. Anterior cervical decompression and arthrodesis for the treatment of cervical spondylotic myelopathy: two to seventeen year follow-up. J Bone Joint Surg Am 1998; 80:941–51.

[53] Emery SE, Bolesta MJ, Banks MA, et al. Robinson anterior cervical fusion: comparison of the standard and modified techniques. Spine 1994;19:660–3.

[54] Cassinelli EH, Hall RA, Kang JD. Biochemistry of intervertebral disc degeneration and the potential for gene therapy applications. Spine J 2001;1:205–14.

implantation, Van Ooij et al [51] found that 67% of these clinical failures had significant subsidence. The investigators believed that subsidence was a significant contributor to poor outcomes after TDR. Of the patients with subsidence, 44% had appropriately sized implants. The mean age of patients with subsidence was 40 years, so it is unlikely that low bone mineral density was responsible for all cases of subsidence. Biomechanical failure of the end plate (subsidence) presents perhaps the most significant challenge to long-term outcomes in TDR. Optimized implant design and end plate coverage may reduce the likelihood of subsidence, but some cases will inevitably occur when today's young arthroplasty patient becomes tomorrow's elderly osteoporotic patient. Therefore, interbody nonfusion implants should be used with caution, particularly in women and patients with risk factors for osteoporosis. Only one case of subsidence of cervical TDR implants has been reported [52]. Longer-term follow-up of these implants is needed to determine whether subsidence will be a clinically significant problem in the cervical spine.

Same level degeneration

The preservation of segmental motion through nonfusion technology introduces the possibility of symptomatic same level degeneration, an entity generally not seen after solid fusion. Potential sources of same level degeneration include the intervertebral disc, the facet joints, and the ligamentum flavum. The intervertebral disc is subject to herniation or painful degeneration after nuclear replacement or posterior stabilization. Preserved motion across facet joints could lead to painful facet arthrosis or stenosis from facet hypertrophy. Finally, ligamentum flavum hypertrophy in the face of preserved intersegmental motion could contribute to stenosis. Same level degeneration has been reported after nonfusion surgery, but its prevalence is difficult to establish. When reported in the literature, same level degeneration is difficult to distinguish from errors in patient selection. For example, a patient who has persistent pain after TDR and requires posterior decompression and fusion may suffer same level degeneration (progression of facet arthrosis) or failure in patient selection (patient had pre-existing stenosis and should have had decompression and fusion as index procedure).

Because segmental motion is retained, progressive facet arthrosis is a clinically significant cause of failure after TDR. Van Ooij et al [51] identified significant facet arthrosis in 41% of patients with failed unconstrained TDR (SB Charité). Lemaire et al [53] noted that some patients had progressive facet arthrosis after unconstrained TDR, but the number of patients was not reported. Huang et al [54] pointed out the importance of biomechanical constraint and neutralization of anterior shear forces in facet preservation. It is possible that constrained implants reduce the incidence of facet arthrosis relative to unconstrained implants. Facet arthrosis that fails nonsurgical treatment can be treated with posterior fusion with implant retention.

Same level disease has also been reported after posterior stabilization. In a series of 82 patients who had implantation of the DYNESYS posterior stabilization system with mean 38-month follow-up, Stoll et al [43] reported that 1 patient (1%) required revision surgery for same level decompression. It is unclear whether the patient had pre-existing stenosis or whether it developed after DYNESYS application. Finally, iatrogenic lateral recess stenosis requiring revision surgery has been reported due to the fixed lordosis that results from Graf ligamentoplasty [55].

Summary

The current evidence on nonfusion implants does not show that these technologies are superior to fusion in mid- to long-term follow-up. Although pseudarthrosis and the need for bone graft are eliminated, it is uncertain whether nonfusion technologies significantly decrease the incidence of adjacent level disease, particularly if segmental motion is not well maintained. Nonfusion implants are subject to a new set of complications including migration, mechanical failure, subsidence, and same level degeneration. The long-term randomized prospective data that are required to accurately weigh the risks and benefits of nonfusion technologies will not be available for many years. Until these long-term data are available, it is difficult to justify widespread adoption of new technologies and abandonment of a "gold standard" (fusion) with a long track record of safety and efficacy. Currently, nonfusion technologies should be reserved for use in a small population of highly selected patients.

References

[1] Wippermann BW, Schratt HE, Steeg S, et al. [Complications of spongiosa harvesting of the ilial crest. A retrospective analysis of 1,191 cases.] Chirurg 1997; 68:1286–91.

[2] Turner JA, Ersek M, Herron L, et al. Patient outcomes after lumbar spinal fusions. JAMA 1992;268:907–11.
[3] Zigler JE, Burd TA, Vialle EN, et al. Lumbar spine arthroplasty: early results using the ProDisc II: a prospective randomized trial of arthroplasty versus fusion. J Spinal Disord Tech 2003;16:352–61.
[4] Delamarter RB, Fribourg DM, Kanim LE, et al. ProDisc artificial total lumbar disc replacement: introduction and early results from the United States clinical trial. Spine 2003;28:S167–75.
[5] Santos ER, Goss DG, Morcom RK, et al. Radiologic assessment of interbody fusion using carbon fiber cages. Spine 2003;28:997–1001.
[6] Whitecloud III TS, Castro Jr FP, Brinker MR, et al. Degenerative conditions of the lumbar spine treated with intervertebral titanium cages and posterior instrumentation for circumferential fusion. J Spinal Disord 1998;11:479–86.
[7] Christensen FB, Hansen ES, Eiskjaer SP, et al. Circumferential lumbar spinal fusion with Brantigan cage versus posterolateral fusion with titanium Cotrel-Dubousset instrumentation: a prospective, randomized clinical study of 146 patients. Spine 2002;27:2674–83.
[8] Fritzell P, Hagg O, Wessberg P, et al. Chronic low back pain and fusion: a comparison of three surgical techniques: a prospective multicenter randomized study from the Swedish lumbar spine study group. Spine 2002;27:1131–41.
[9] Madan S, Boeree NR. Outcome of posterior lumbar interbody fusion versus posterolateral fusion for spondylolytic spondylolisthesis. Spine 2002;27:1536–42.
[10] Thalgott JS, Klezl Z, Timlin M, et al. Anterior lumbar interbody fusion with processed sea coral (coralline hydroxyapatite) as part of a circumferential fusion. Spine 2002;27:E518–25 [discussion: E26–7].
[11] Moore KR, Pinto MR, Butler LM. Degenerative disc disease treated with combined anterior and posterior arthrodesis and posterior instrumentation. Spine 2002;27:1680–6.
[12] Liljenqvist U, O'Brien JP, Renton P. Simultaneous combined anterior and posterior lumbar fusion with femoral cortical allograft. Eur Spine J 1998;7:125–31.
[13] Barnes B, Rodts GE, McLaughlin MR, et al. Threaded cortical bone dowels for lumbar interbody fusion: over 1-year mean follow up in 28 patients. J Neurosurg 2001;95:1–4.
[14] Loguidice VA, Johnson RG, Guyer RD, et al. Anterior lumbar interbody fusion. Spine 1988;13:366–9.
[15] Sasso RC, Kitchel SH, Dawson EG. A prospective, randomized controlled clinical trial of anterior lumbar interbody fusion using a titanium cylindrical threaded fusion device. Spine 2004;29:113–22 [discussion: 21–2].
[16] Thalgott JS, Fritts K, Giuffre JM, et al. Anterior interbody fusion of the cervical spine with coralline hydroxyapatite. Spine 1999;24:1295–9.
[17] Bohlman HH, Emery SE, Goodfellow DB, et al. Robinson anterior cervical discectomy and arthrodesis for cervical radiculopathy. Long-term follow-up of one hundred and twenty-two patients. J Bone Joint Surg Am 1993;75:1298–307.
[18] Emery SE, Fisher JR, Bohlman HH. Three-level anterior cervical discectomy and fusion: radiographic and clinical results. Spine 1997;22:2622–4 [discussion: 5].
[19] Bolesta MJ, Rechtine II GR, Chrin AM. Three- and four-level anterior cervical discectomy and fusion with plate fixation: a prospective study. Spine 2000;25:2040–4 [discussion: 5–6].
[20] Wang JC, McDonough PW, Kanim LE, et al. Increased fusion rates with cervical plating for three-level anterior cervical discectomy and fusion. Spine 2001;26:643–6 [discussion: 6–7].
[21] Kornblum MB, Fischgrund JS, Herkowitz HN, et al. Degenerative lumbar spondylolisthesis with spinal stenosis: a prospective long-term study comparing fusion and pseudarthrosis. Spine 2004;29:726–33 [discussion: 33–4].
[22] Phillips FM, Carlson G, Emery SE, et al. Anterior cervical pseudarthrosis. Natural history and treatment. Spine 1997;22:1585–9.
[23] Newman M. The outcome of pseudarthrosis after cervical anterior fusion. Spine 1993;18:2380–2.
[24] Penta M, Sandhu A, Fraser RD. Magnetic resonance imaging assessment of disc degeneration 10 years after anterior lumbar interbody fusion. Spine 1995;20:743–7.
[25] Rahm MD, Hall BB. Adjacent-segment degeneration after lumbar fusion with instrumentation: a retrospective study. J Spinal Disord 1996;9:392–400.
[26] Leong JC, Chun SY, Grange WJ, et al. Long-term results of lumbar intervertebral disc prolapse. Spine 1983;8:793–9.
[27] Kumar MN, Jacquot F, Hall H. Long-term follow-up of functional outcomes and radiographic changes at adjacent levels following lumbar spine fusion for degenerative disc disease. Eur Spine J 2001;10:309–13.
[28] Ishihara H, Osada R, Kanamori M, et al. Minimum 10-year follow-up study of anterior lumbar interbody fusion for isthmic spondylolisthesis. J Spinal Disord 2001;14:91–9.
[29] Miyakoshi N, Abe E, Shimada Y, et al. Outcome of one-level posterior lumbar interbody fusion for spondylolisthesis and postoperative intervertebral disc degeneration adjacent to the fusion. Spine 2000;25:1837–42.
[30] Ghiselli G, Wang JC, Bhatia NN, et al. Adjacent segment degeneration in the lumbar spine. J Bone Joint Surg Am 2004;86:1497–503.
[31] Hilibrand AS, Carlson GD, Palumbo MA, et al. Radiculopathy and myelopathy at segments adjacent to the site of a previous anterior cervical arthrodesis. J Bone Joint Surg Am 1999;81:519–28.
[32] Boden SD, Davis DO, Dina TS, et al. Abnormal magnetic-resonance scans of the lumbar spine in asymptomatic subjects. A prospective investigation. J Bone Joint Surg Am 1990;72:403–8.
[33] Boden SD, McCowin PR, Davis DO, et al. Abnormal

magnetic-resonance scans of the cervical spine in asymptomatic subjects. A prospective investigation. J Bone Joint Surg Am 1990;72:1178–84.
[34] Chou WY, Hsu CJ, Chang WN, et al. Adjacent segment degeneration after lumbar spinal posterolateral fusion with instrumentation in elderly patients. Arch Orthop Trauma Surg 2002;122:39–43.
[35] Whitecloud III TS, Davis JM, Olive PM. Operative treatment of the degenerated segment adjacent to a lumbar fusion. Spine 1994;19:531–6.
[36] Schlegel JD, Smith JA, Schleusener RL. Lumbar motion segment pathology adjacent to thoracolumbar, lumbar, and lumbosacral fusions. Spine 1996;21: 970–81.
[37] Lee CK. Accelerated degeneration of the segment adjacent to a lumbar fusion. Spine 1988;13:375–7.
[38] Glassman SD, Pugh K, Johnson JR, et al. Surgical management of adjacent level degeneration following lumbar spine fusion. Orthopedics 2002;25:1051–5.
[39] Kanayama M, Hashimoto T, Shigenobu K, et al. Adjacent-segment morbidity after Graf ligamentoplasty compared with posterolateral lumbar fusion. J Neurosurg 2001;95:5–10.
[40] Huang RC, Girardi FP, Cammisa Jr FP, et al. Long-term flexion-extension range of motion of the prodisc total disc replacement. J Spinal Disord Tech 2003;16: 435–40.
[41] Huang RC, Girardi FP, Cammisa Jr FP, et al. The relationship between range of motion and outcome in lumbar total disc replacement at 9-year follow-up. Presented at the 19th Annual Meeting of the North American Spine Society. Chicago, 2004.
[42] Huang RC, Girardi FP, Lim MR, et al. Range of motion and adjacent level degeneration after lumbar total disc replacement. Presented at the 39th Annual Meeting of the Scoliosis Research Society. Buenos Aires, Argentina, 2004.
[43] Stoll TM, Dubois G, Schwarzenbach O. The dynamic neutralization system for the spine: a multi-center study of a novel non-fusion system. Eur Spine J 2002; 11(Suppl 2):S170–8.
[44] Kuslich SD, Danielson G, Dowdle JD, et al. Four-year follow-up results of lumbar spine arthrodesis using the Bagby and Kuslich lumbar fusion cage. Spine 2000; 25:2656–62.
[45] Schmoelz W, Huber JF, Nydegger T, et al. Dynamic stabilization of the lumbar spine and its effects on adjacent segments: an in vitro experiment. J Spinal Disord Tech 2003;16:418–23.
[46] Szpalski M, Gunzburg R, Mayer M. Spine arthroplasty: a historical review. Eur Spine J 2002;11(Suppl 2): S65–84.
[47] Griffith SL, Shelokov AP, Buttner-Janz K, et al. A multicenter retrospective study of the clinical results of the LINK SB Charite intervertebral prosthesis. The initial European experience. Spine 1994;19:1842–9.
[48] Mayer HM, Wiechert K, Korge A, Qose I. Minimally invasive total disc replacement: surgical technique and preliminary clinical results. Eur Spine J 2002; 11(Suppl 2):S124–30.
[49] Bertagnoli R, Schonmayr R. Surgical and clinical results with the PDN prosthetic disc-nucleus device. Eur Spine J 2002;11(Suppl 2):S143–8.
[50] Cinotti G, David T, Postacchini F. Results of disc prosthesis after a minimum follow-up period of 2 years. Spine 1996;21:995–1000.
[51] Van Ooij A, Oner FC, Verbout AJ. Complications of artificial disc replacement: a report of 27 patients with the SB Charite disc. J Spinal Disord Tech 2003;16: 369–83.
[52] Wigfield CC, Gill SS, Nelson RJ, et al. The new Frenchay artificial cervical joint: results from a two-year pilot study. Spine 2002;27:2446–52.
[53] Lemaire JP, Skalli W, Lavaste F, et al. Intervertebral disc prosthesis. Results and prospects for the year 2000. Clin Orthop 1997;337:64–76.
[54] Huang RC, Girardi FP, Cammisa Jr FP, et al. The implications of constraint in lumbar total disc replacement. J Spinal Disord Tech 2003;16:412–7.
[55] Mulholland RC, Sengupta DK. Rationale, principles and experimental evaluation of the concept of soft stabilization. Eur Spine J 2002;11(Suppl 2):S198–205.

Biomechanics of Nonfusion Implants

Russel C. Huang, MD[a,b,*], Timothy M. Wright, PhD[b,c],
Manohar M. Panjabi, PhD, DTech[d], Joseph D. Lipman, MS[b,c]

[a]*Hospital for Special Surgery, 535 East 70th Street, New York, NY 10021, USA*
[b]*Weill Cornell Medical College, New York, NY, USA*
[c]*Laboratory for Biomedical Mechanics, Hospital for Special Surgery, 535 East 70th Street, New York, NY 10021, USA*
[d]*Biomechanics Laboratory, Department of Orthopaedics and Rehabilitation, Yale University School of Medicine, 367 Cedar Street, New Haven, CT 06510, USA*

Spine fusion is a versatile and effective tool in the management of a wide variety of spinal instabilities, deformities, and painful conditions. A growing body of biomechanical and clinical evidence, however, suggests that the relative immobility of fused spinal segments transfers stress to adjacent segments, leading to acceleration of adjacent level degeneration. Furthermore, the sagittal alignment of a fused spinal segment is fixed and cannot adapt to variations in posture. Nonfusion technologies in spine surgery are being developed to address these perceived shortcomings of fusion. In this article, the authors review the relevant biomechanics of the functional spinal unit (FSU) in health and disease and the biomechanical design concepts behind several classes of nonfusion implants.

The normal functional spinal unit

Anatomy and spinal loading

The spinal motion segments are exquisitely designed to provide a remarkable combination of stability, mobility, and load transmission. The primary load-bearing and stabilizing structure of the FSU is the intervertebral disc. The outer anulus fibrosus is composed of concentric lamellae of fibrocartilaginous and fibrous connective tissue oriented in an alternating pattern analogous to that of a radial tire [1]. Its structure makes the anulus ideally suited to bear the tensile hoop stresses that result from pressurization of the intact nucleus pulposus. The nucleus pulposus is located in the posterocentral area of the disc and is composed primarily of proteoglycans suspended in a loosely organized collagen network. The hydrophilic nature of proteoglycans is responsible for the maintenance of disc turgor and makes the nucleus well suited to bear and redistribute compressive loads. To extend the automobile tire analogy, the turgid nucleus acts as the air within the tire. With sufficient turgor, compressive loads on the incompressible nucleus are redistributed radially, creating tensile loads in the anulus fibrosus. The collagen fibers of the anulus are well suited to bear tensile loads. As a mechanical structure, the healthy nucleus pulposus is relatively isotropic, and loads are therefore distributed evenly to the underlying end plate (Fig. 1) [2].

Facet joints provide secondary load-bearing and stabilizing functions in the FSU. Their anatomy varies widely by spinal region and determines their specific biomechanical function [3]. In the cervical spine, the orientation of the facets is approximated by a plane midway between the coronal and axial planes. Due to their orientation, cervical facet joints are the primary restraint to anterior translation of the cephalad vertebra with anterior shear loading and provide significant resistance to extension [4]. Thus, facet cartilage is loaded by anterior shear forces during extension.

* Corresponding author. Hospital for Special Surgery, 535 East 70th Street, New York, NY 10021.
E-mail address: huangr@hss.edu (R.C. Huang).

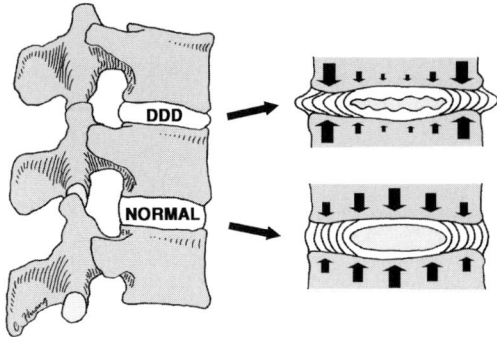

Fig. 1. Load transfer in normal and degenerated (DDD) discs. Note uniform load transmission across disc space in normal, relatively isotropic disc. In degenerated disc, the nucleus pulposus has lost turgor and therefore its ability to transmit load. Therefore, load is transferred across peripheral region of disc space by annular tissue.

In the lumbar spine, facet orientation can be approximated by a plane located midway between the sagittal and coronal planes that is slightly inclined anteriorly. Lumbar facet joints provide resistance to excessive extension but experience high compressive loads in extension. In contrast, they experience minimal loads in flexion or compression loading of the spine. Anterior shear loads also increase facet pressures [5]. In posterior shear loading, facets are unloaded, but the posterior ligaments (supraspinous, interspinous, facet capsules) resist posterior translation and are subjected to tensile loads [5,6]. Facet loads are large [7], which is clinically relevant because the facets are known pain generators in the lumbar spine [8,9].

The spine's ability to bear large loads in compression, shear, and torsion while providing motion and stability to the spinal column is truly impressive. Physiologic loads in the lumbar spine are substantial and repetitive, and nonfusion implants must therefore be able to bear high cyclic loads for many decades. Compressive loads on lumbar intervertebral discs are 1.0 to 2.5 times body weight during normal walking [10]. During the lifting of 14- to 27-kg objects, axial compressive loads in the lumbar spine are estimated to be 5300 to 6900 N (7.6 to 9.9 times body weight for a 70-kg person) and anteroposterior shear loads are estimated to range from 1100 to 1500 N (1.6 to 2.1 times body weight) [11]. Anteroposterior shear loads reach 700 N during trunk extension at 70% of maximal torque generation [12]. Approximately 80% of compressive loads applied to the spine pass through the anterior column of the lumbar spine; the remainder are transmitted by the facets [13,14]. Degeneration of the intervertebral disc, loss of disc height, or alterations in sagittal alignment, however, may result in greater load transfer to facet joints.

Kinematics

The kinematics of an FSU describe the arcs of motion that the two vertebral bodies follow during movement of the spine. Although motions in different planes are often coupled, kinematics can be described more simply by considering movements to be combinations of flexion–extension, lateral bending, and axial rotation and then by considering these rotations separately. The flexion–extension instantaneous axis of rotation (IAR) of a cervical or lumbar motion segment can be approximated by a point slightly posterior and distal to the center of the inferior vertebral end plate. The precise location of the IAR depends on the level in the spine and migrates during intervertebral motion [15–17]. In the lumbar spine, L5-S1 is a notable exception because the IAR lies within the disc space instead of below the inferior end plate. Moving from C2 to C7, the IAR likewise moves proximally, lying closer to the disc space in more distal levels. Because the posterior elements move in concert with the anterior elements, and because the posterior elements have complex three-dimensional topography, the changes in kinematics caused by significant perturbation of the normal IAR can result in excessive facet joint or posterior ligamentous loading. This factor is important to consider in the design of nonfusion implants.

The magnitude of FSU motions varies widely between different levels of the spine and between individuals [18]. In general, mean flexion–extension range of motion ranges from 10° to 20° per level in the cervical spine and from 9° to 14° per level in the lumbar spine. Nonfusion implants should be designed to accommodate ranges of motion similar to normal FSUs. Nonphysiologic motion could contribute to same-level degeneration by way of facet arthrosis and hypertrophy, ligamentum flavum hypertrophy, or disc degeneration. On the other hand, implants with inadequate motion may not reduce the incidence of adjacent level disease, one of the primary goals of nonfusion technology.

The diseased functional spinal unit

Uniform distribution of compressive loads across the disc space and the maintenance of tensile loading of the anulus are dependent on nuclear turgor.

The degenerated disc with loss of nuclear hydration has been likened to a flat tire. In the degenerated motion segment, the nucleus loses its ability to bear compressive loads and load transfer shifts to the anulus, a structure that is poorly suited to withstand compression. In addition, loading with inadequate nuclear turgor leads to shearing forces in the transitional zone between the nucleus and anulus, causing fatigue failure, fissuring, and further degeneration. As the mechanical integrity of the nucleus deteriorates, its isotropic load transfer properties are lost; instead, load transfer is concentrated at the periphery (annular insertion) of the vertebral end plates (see Fig. 1). The loss of disc hydration and turgor is one of the initiating steps in the degenerative cascade that culminates in diffuse disc and facet degeneration.

Degenerative changes in the intervertebral disc can lead to progressive facet arthrosis. Early and intermediate stages of degenerative disc disease lead to relative disc laxity [19,20]. As the degenerating disc becomes less able to resist rotations and shear, additional stresses are transferred to the posterior elements. Pain from degenerative disc disease may arise from compressed neural structures, degenerated facets [8], the disc itself [21], or from the eccentrically loaded vertebral end plate [22,23]. Most clinicians agree that the symptomatic degenerated segment with advanced anterior and posterior element disease is best treated with fusion, although this consensus may change as the indications and contraindications for nonfusion technology evolve [24,25].

Biomechanics of fused segments

Cadaveric studies [13,26,27], finite element analyses [28,29], and animal studies [30] have demonstrated that fusion increases intradiscal pressures, end plate stresses, and annular stresses at adjacent segments. In clinical practice, adjacent level degeneration after fusion is frequently encountered [31–34]. Adjacent level degeneration is thought to result primarily from increased motion and stress at adjacent levels because of the restricted motion across the fused segments. In addition, the fixed sagittal alignment of fused segments cannot accommodate regional alignment changes that occur in sitting, supine, and erect postures. Fused segments in suboptimal sagittal alignment have been linked to the development of adjacent level degeneration [35–37]. The precise incidence rate and clinical impact of adjacent level disease are difficult to define, but it is clearly a common long-term complication of an otherwise successful arthrodesis and its avoidance is one of the driving forces behind the development of nonfusion technologies.

Biomechanics of total disc replacement

The underlying basis for total disc replacement (TDR) is the same as that of total joint replacement of the hip or knee. Elimination of the painful degenerated disc, like the degenerated articular cartilage in an arthritic hip or knee, relieves pain. Furthermore, maintenance of segmental motion may reduce the incidence of adjacent level degeneration and allows the implanted segment to adjust its sagittal alignment to accommodate functional demands. Because motion is preserved and only anterior column pathology is addressed, TDR is contraindicated in patients with pre-existing facet arthrosis. Assuming that load transmission through the TDR implant (instead of the intervertebral disc) eliminates the disc as a pain generator, the performance of a TDR will depend on four design objectives. First, the implant should perform under physiologic cyclic loading conditions for a period of at least 5 decades without experiencing mechanical or wear-related failure. Second, the implant's kinematics should not lead to progressive facet arthrosis at the implanted level. Third, the implant should retain enough motion to reduce the development of adjacent level degeneration. Finally, the fixation and footprint of the implant should be optimized to reduce the incidence of subsidence and loosening. The performance of a TDR implant that does not meet all of these criteria may be inferior to that of fusion in the long-term.

The average hip arthroplasty patient completes 2 million walking cycles per year [38]. Taking into account the 6 million smaller motions associated with respiration over a year, a typical FSU undergoes approximately 8 million motion cycles per year. By heeding the lessons learned on orthopedic implant durability over the last 30 years, it should be possible to design TDR implants with low rates of mechanical failure. For example, early versions of the SB Charité implant (Depuy Spine, Raynham, Massachussetts) suffered high rates of metallic end plate fatigue fracture [39], but design and metallurgic improvements have virtually eliminated this complication. In contrast to hip and knee arthroplasty, polyethylene wear has not been a prominent problem thus far in lumbar TDR. The first-generation Charité implants were placed in the early 1980s, and no histologically confirmed cases of osteolysis have been reported in the literature. Cinotti et al [40] and Tropiano et al [41] were unable to detect loss of polyethylene thickness by plain radiographs at 2-year and 9-year follow-up, respectively. Alternative bearings such as metal-on-metal, ceramic-on-polyethylene, and ceramic-on-ceramic—all of which have shown promise in total

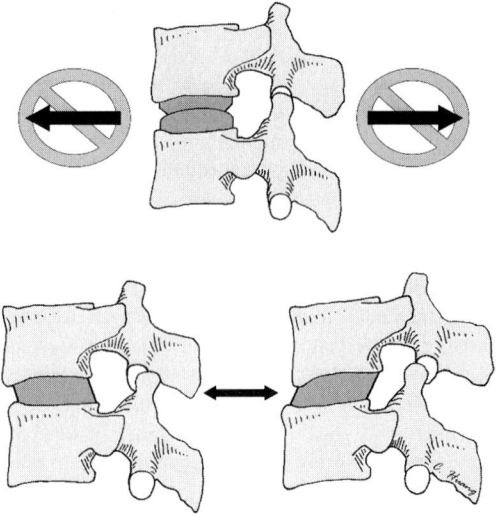

Fig. 2. With constrained ball-and-socket implant (*above*), pure anteroposterior translations (shear) are prohibited provided the ball-and-socket remains coapted. With less constrained implants (*below*), anteroposterior shear forces are absorbed by facet joints instead of the implant.

or lateral translational intervertebral motion. A constrained TDR is typified by the ball-and-socket articulation of the ProDisc (Synthes-Stratec, Paoli, Pennsylvania), Maverick (Medtronic Sofamor Danek, Memphis, Tennessee), or Prestige (Medtronic Sofamor Danek) implants. The SB Charité, which allows a small amount of shear translation, is a less constrained implant.

In the cervical and lumbar spine, facet cartilage tends to be loaded by anterior shear loads. Constrained implants are able to neutralize anterior shear loads and thereby reduce loading of the facets but do so at the expense of greater loads on the implant and the implant–bone interface. In contrast, implants with less constraint to anterior-posterior shear may allow increased facet loading (Fig. 2). Finally, because a constrained TDR dictates the arc of rotation followed by the FSU, to the extent that the motion arc dictated by the implant is inappropriate for the three-dimensional topography of the posterior elements, a constrained implant may cause high facet loading at extremes of motion.

For implants with congruent spherical bearing surfaces (such as ball-and-socket TDRs), kinematic properties are determined largely by the location of the IAR and the radius of curvature of the articulation. The IAR is the point in space around which the cephalad component and its attached vertebral body rotate. The radius of curvature is the distance from the IAR to the implant's bearing surface. Essentially, implants with a large radius of curvature appear "flat" and those with a small radius of curvature appear "round." Although apparent translation of the vertebral body occurs during motion of constrained ball-and-socket implants, this motion is in fact rotation of the vertebral body around the implant's IAR (Fig. 3). The relative proportion of rotation and apparent translation observed in a ball-

hip arthroplasty—may also provide good longevity in spine arthroplasty. Although lumbar loads are large, rotations and other motions are small in comparison to hip and knee joints. Because abrasive and adhesive wear are a function of load and sliding distance, wear and the associated particle-induced osteolysis may not be significant problems in TDR.

The use of viscoelastic materials in load-bearing environments, particularly where shear loads are also applied, has not been as successful as the use of "hard" bearings. Silicone implants have been plagued by high rates of fragmentation and failure when used for arthroplasty of the hand, foot, wrist, or elbow [42–45]. The Acroflex lumbar TDR (Acromed Corp., Cleveland, Ohio), which was made with a vulcanized rubber core, had unacceptably high rates of mechanical failure [46]. Implant designers should use viscoelastic materials with caution in locations subject to repetitive compressive, torsion, and shear loading.

Because anterior pain-generating structures have been ablated or unloaded by TDR, long-term results may be strongly influenced by long-term preservation of the facet joints. Biomechanical constraint and kinematics of a TDR implant affect the facet joints. The implications of biomechanical constraint and other implant design characteristics in facet preservation after lumbar TDR were reviewed by Huang et al [47]. For the purposes of TDR, constraint can be defined as the limitation of pure anteroposterior

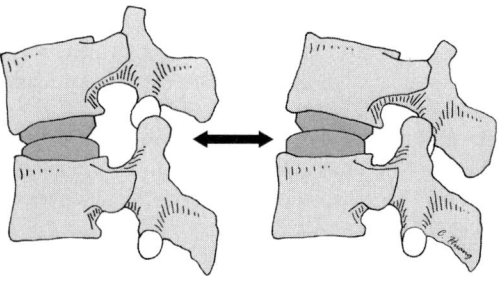

Fig. 3. Although apparent anteroposterior translation of the cephalad vertebra occurs with motion of a constrained implant, this motion is in fact rotation around the implant's IAR.

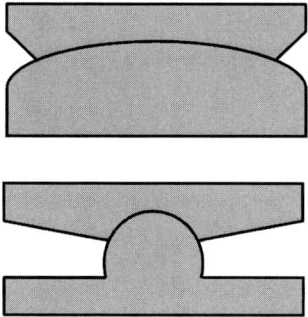

Fig. 4. With a ball-and socket articulation, the relative proportion of rotational and apparent translational motions depends on the radius of curvature. "Round" implants (*below*) are rotation dominant, whereas in "flat" implants (*above*), apparent translation dominates.

and-socket TDR is determined by the radius of curvature of the implant. With a small (round) radius of curvature, rotation dominates. With a large (flat) radius of curvature, translation dominates (Fig. 4).

The effects of different kinematic patterns on facet loads can be predicted based on facet joint anatomy. In general, extension tends to load facets, whereas flexion unloads them. Anterior translation tends to load facets, and posterior translation unloads them. Although preservation of flexion–extension motion is important in reducing stresses on adjacent levels, the interplay of flexion–extension rotations and translational motion affects facet loading. Implant designers should consider these factors when specifying the degree of constraint, the location of the IAR, and the radius of curvature of TDRs.

Because preserved rotation at the affected FSU reduces stresses on adjacent levels, the magnitude of TDR motion will likely affect long-term outcome. Although most short-term studies document near-physiologic prosthetic motion, the magnitude of TDR motion may decrease with time. Most short-term (<5 years) radiographic studies of constrained and unconstrained lumbar TDR implants demonstrate flexion–extension rotations on the order of 10° [40,48–50]. Short-term follow-up of cervical TDR demonstrated mean retained motion of 7° to 11° [51–53]. Nine-year follow-up of the ProDisc first-generation implant, however, demonstrated mean motion of only 3.8°, with 34% of the implants having less than 2° of motion [54]. A recent report of mean 17-year follow-up of the SB Charité implant revealed that 59% of implants had no measurable motion on radiographs [55]. Therefore, a significant number of TDRs become kinematically equivalent to a fusion over time; nonetheless, some patients retain significant motion, which may improve outcomes compared with fusion. Reviewing 9-year follow-up data of the ProDisc first-generation implant, Huang et al [54,56] found that TDR patients with a low range of motion had increased adjacent level degeneration [54] and inferior clinical outcome [56]. Motion of at least 5° conferred a significant advantage in clinical outcomes and reduction in adjacent level degeneration [57]. Studies on TDR motion have focused on flexion–extension motion. Lateral bending and axial rotation may also be significant factors affecting outcome but are difficult to measure because the rotations are of such small magnitude.

The same design factors that affect facet loading influence the rotational range of motion achieved by a TDR implant [47]. These factors include the anteroposterior location of the IAR, the radius of curvature, the height, and the amount of constraint of the implant. A relatively posterior IAR better reflects the physiologic IAR and results in greater range of motion [58]. A larger radius of curvature in a ball-and-socket TDR reduces the amount of rotation achieved by a TDR. Assuming that coaptation of bearing surfaces is maintained, a constrained TDR dictates the arc of rotation followed by the FSU. The more the arc dictated by the implant is resisted by the anatomy of the posterior elements, the more the resulting motion is restricted. Although no disc implant can perfectly replicate the kinematics of a normal disc, the design of TDR implants can be optimized by selecting a level of constraint, a location of IAR, and a radius of curvature that is appropriate for the FSU in question. The ideal implant characteristics will vary between levels and between individuals.

Subsidence of TDR implants has been observed in up to 67% of clinically failed lumbar TDRs [48]. The occurrence of subsidence after TDR is not surprising given the compliance mismatch between a metallic implant and the adjacent vertebral end plate and vertebral cancellous bone. Normal age-related declines in bone mineral density will exacerbate this mismatch over time in most patients. In contrast to a TDR implant, an interbody fusion mass has the ability to remodel and would be expected to match the compliance of the adjacent vertebral bodies.

Although it is inevitable that some TDR patients will experience significant subsidence, its incidence may be reduced by attention to surgical technique and implant design. Because an ossified remnant of the ring apophysis remains in adulthood, the peripheral rim of the vertebral end plate is thicker than the central area. Because load transfer in degenerated discs with insufficient turgor is shifted peripherally to the anulus, the relative strength advantage of the peripheral end plate may be even more pronounced in degenerative disc disease. Numerous investigators have pointed out the importance of seating interbody implants on this thickened peripheral ring of bone [59]. This principle should also be applied to TDR implants. Anatomic designs with maximized end plate coverage may also reduce the incidence of subsidence. In the lumbar spine, the end plates are thickest in the posterolateral aspects of the rim [60]. In the cervical spine, superior end plates are thicker posteriorly, whereas inferior end plates are thicker anteriorly [61]. Thinning of the end plates with burs or other instruments should be minimized.

The effect of adjuvant fixation structures such as keels, pegs, or teeth penetrating the end plate and extending from the metallic plate into the underlying cancellous bone have not been studied in the vertebra to the authors' knowledge. Finally, because women generally have greater loss of bone mineral density with age and therefore increased susceptibility to subsidence, TDRs should be implanted with caution in women regardless of design.

Biomechanics of nuclear implants

Nucleus pulposus implants are designed to re-establish more normal disc function by restoring disc turgor, tension in the anulus fibrosus, and the disc's ability to transfer loads uniformly across the disc space. Most designs use viscoelastic polymers that are preformed or injected into the disc space in monomer form and polymerize in situ. The only implant with significant clinical experience to date is the Prosthetic Disc Nucleus (PDN; RAYMEDICA, Bloomington, Minnesota). The PDN is composed of a hydrogel pellet encased in a woven polyethylene jacket. PDN devices are inserted through a posterolateral or lateral annulotomy in a dehydrated state. The hydrogel imbibes water, expanding in volume and theoretically re-establishing nuclear function by restoring disc turgor.

Because prosthetic nuclear replacements are designed to re-tension the anulus, a relatively competent anulus fibrosus is required. Large annular defects and advanced vertical disc space collapse are contraindications to nucleus replacement. Clinical experience has shown that the PDN provides sustained increases in disc space height at 2- to 4-year follow-up [62,63]. Because compressive lumbar loads during activities of daily living are so large [11], it is not surprising that some implants have had significant extrusion rates. Design changes to render implants less able to extrude through annular defects and implantation through lateral instead of posterolateral annulotomies have significantly decreased the rate of extrusion [63].

End plate remodeling has been observed after implantation of the PDN. Areas of end plate sclerosis are probably a response to concentrated load transfer through the device, which does not cover the entire end plate and therefore cannot restore the uniform load distribution properties of the healthy intervertebral disc. If it is painless and if disc height is maintained, then end plate remodeling may be of no clinical significance; however, cases with severe remodeling and loss of height have been reported [63]. In response to this phenomenon, the PDN device was altered to increase its water content to increase its compliance. Maximizing end plate coverage and minimizing implant stiffness should reduce the incidence of end plate remodeling.

Randomized trials are required to establish the efficacy of nucleus pulposus replacement. Furthermore, longer follow-up periods are required to ensure that nuclear replacements are not susceptible to fatigue failure given the large magnitude of lumbar spine loads during activities of daily living.

Biomechanics of posterior stabilization devices

In contrast to the principles of TDR, whereby painful disc tissues are ablated or unloaded directly by the implant, posterior stabilization devices leave the pain-generating disc tissues in situ but restrict certain types of motion and alter load transfer through the FSU. In addition, some implants are designed to unload the disc and facets by load sharing. The properties of currently available and proposed soft stabilization devices were reviewed in detail by Mulholland et al [64] and Sengupta [65]. The soft stabilization device with the most clinical experience is the Graf (SEM Co., Montrouge, France) ligamentoplasty. The implant consists of titanium pedicle screws connected by prosthetic ligaments that are tensioned to hold the FSU in lordosis. The implant's inventor believed that painful lumbar instability resulted from pathologic facet distraction and subluxation occurring during axial rotation [66]. The implant is intended to maintain lordotic apposition of the facet joints and to eliminate the pathologic motion. Although it was first developed for the treatment of back pain resulting from disc degeneration in the setting of preserved posterior elements [67–70], it has also been used to stabilize spondylolisthetic motion segments following posterior decompression [71].

Because the FSU is fixed in lordosis, unloading of the anterior disc occurs with load transfer to the posterior anulus and facets. Essentially, the posterior anulus acts as a fulcrum between the tensile forces applied posteriorly by the Graf device and the compressive forces applied across the disc space. Overloading of the posterior anulus is a theoretic concern, but encouragingly, no progressive loss of posterior disc height has been detected at a mean of 3.4 years of follow-up [72]. The other potential problem resulting from forced extension is the development of iatrogenic lateral recess stenosis [69].

The DYNESYS system (Zimmer, Warsaw, Indiana) is similar to the Graf system, with the addition of compression-resistant polycarbonate urethane sleeves around the prosthetic ligaments (Fig. 5). The motion segment can be stabilized in a more neutral alignment instead of lordosis. The prosthetic ligaments provide restraint to flexion, whereas the sleeves prevent excessive lordosis, bear compressive loads, and unload the disc when the patient's musculature exerts a net lordotic moment on the FSU. With kyphotic moments, the prosthetic ligaments prevent excessive motion. With lordotic moments, the plastic sleeves assume some load-bearing function. Although overload of the posterior anulus may be avoided, three potential problems are introduced by the DYNESYS system. First, the compressive sleeves limit the amount of lordosis that can be achieved, and if placed with excessive distraction, the implant becomes kyphogenic. Second, compressive loads on the sleeves produce bending moments on the pedicle screws that could lead to breakage or loosening.

In fact, Stoll et al [73] reported that 10% of patients (7/73) had radiographically evident DYNESYS screw loosening at a mean of 38 months of follow-up, whereas screw loosening after Graf ligamentoplasty has not been widely reported. Third, the introduction of compression sleeves significantly increases the rigidity of the construct. The retained motion of the Graf system has been reported as a mean of 4.3° at 31-month follow-up [67]. Biomechanical testing has shown that in flexion–extension and lateral bending, the kinematics of a motion segment stabilized by DYNESYS are statistically indistinguishable from those of a rigidly instrumented motion segment [74]. It is doubtful that the incidence of adjacent level degeneration would be decreased by such a rigid construct.

Posterior stabilization devices may be susceptible to fatigue failure from cyclic loading. For many types of orthopedic implants including total hip and knee arthroplasty components, the repetitive loads placed on the implant by the patient are below the endurance limit of the metallic alloys used to fabricate the components, and fatigue failure is therefore rarely observed. This is not the case with pedicle screw instrumentation, which is subject to fatigue failure with prolonged cyclic loading in cases of failed arthrodesis. Because arthrodesis is not performed when implanting posterior stabilization devices, fatigue failure may occur after time. In addition, the polymers used to manufacture prosthetic ligaments and compression-bearing sleeves (as in the DYNESYS system) may fail due to fatigue or wear.

Summary

The FSU's ability to provide mobility and stability over many decades while withstanding repetitive application of high loads in multiple planes is truly impressive. In many patients, however, degenerative diseases of the spine eventually cause significant pain and disability. Fusion remains one of the most useful and versatile tools in the spine surgeon's armamentarium but is not without shortcomings. The development of nonfusion implants that can relieve pain, restore motion, and endure repetitive loads and the healthy motion segment is a daunting challenge. The design of optimized implants requires understanding of the pathophysiology of spinal pain syndromes, vertebral macro- and microanatomy, motion segment kinematics, and loads applied to spine. In addition, adherence to sound engineering principles and knowledge of materials science are essential.

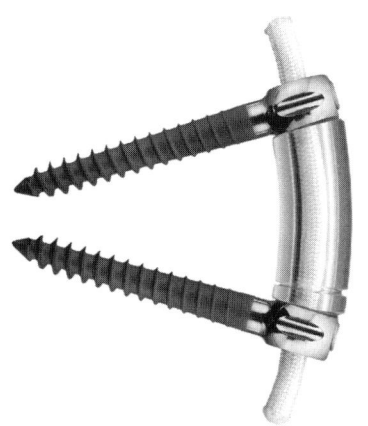

Fig. 5. DYNESYS pedicle screws, prosthetic ligament, and compression sleeve. (Courtesy of Zimmer Spine, Inc., Minneapolis, Minnesota; with permission.)

Acknowledgments

The authors gratefully acknowledge the illustrations provided by Chi-Ming C. Huang.

References

[1] Hickey DS, Hukins DW. X-ray diffraction studies of the arrangement of collagenous fibres in human fetal intervertebral disc. J Anat 1980;131:81–90.

[2] Hukins DW. A simple model for the function of proteoglycans and collagen in the response to compression of the intervertebral disc. Proc R Soc Lond B Biol Sci 1992;249:281–5.

[3] Panjabi MM, Oxland T, Takata K, et al. Articular facets of the human spine. Quantitative three-dimensional anatomy. Spine 1993;18:1298–310.

[4] Ng HW, Teo EC, Lee KK, et al. Finite element analysis of cervical spinal instability under physiologic loading. J Spinal Disord Tech 2003;16:55–65.

[5] Sharma M, Langrana NA, Rodriguez J. Role of ligaments and facets in lumbar spinal stability. Spine 1995;20:887–900.

[6] Sharma M, Langrana NA, Rodriguez J. Modeling of facet articulation as a nonlinear moving contact problem: sensitivity study on lumbar facet response. J Biomech Eng 1998;120:118–25.

[7] Schendel MJ, Wood KB, Buttermann GR, et al. Experimental measurement of ligament force, facet force, and segment motion in the human lumbar spine. J Biomech 1993;26:427–38.

[8] Dreyer SJ, Dreyfuss PH. Low back pain and the zygapophysial (facet) joints. Arch Phys Med Rehabil 1996;77:290–300.

[9] Cavanaugh JM, Ozaktay AC, Yamashita HT, et al. Lumbar facet pain: biomechanics, neuroanatomy and neurophysiology. J Biomech 1996;29:1117–29.

[10] Cappozzo A. Compressive loads in the lumbar vertebral column during normal level walking. J Orthop Res 1984;1:292–301.

[11] Granata KP, Marras WS, Davis KG. Variation in spinal load and trunk dynamics during repeated lifting exertions. Clin Biomech (Bristol, Avon) 1999;14:367–75.

[12] Sparto PJ, Parnianpour M. Estimation of trunk muscle forces and spinal loads during fatiguing repetitive trunk exertions. Spine 1998;23:2563–73.

[13] Cunningham BW, Kotani Y, McNulty PS, et al. The effect of spinal destabilization and instrumentation on lumbar intradiscal pressure: an in vitro biomechanical analysis. Spine 1997;22:2655–63.

[14] Bergmark A. Stability of the lumbar spine. A study in mechanical engineering. Acta Orthop Scand Suppl 1989;230:1–54.

[15] Gertzbein SD, Holtby R, Tile M, et al. Determination of a locus of instantaneous centers of rotation of the lumbar disc by moire fringes. A new technique. Spine 1984;9:409–13.

[16] Pearcy MJ, Bogduk N. Instantaneous axes of rotation of the lumbar intervertebral joints. Spine 1988;13:1033–41.

[17] Yoshioka T, Tsuji H, Hirano N, et al. Motion characteristic of the normal lumbar spine in young adults: instantaneous axis of rotation and vertebral center motion analyses. J Spinal Disord 1990;3:103–13.

[18] Hayes MA, Howard TC, Gruel CR, et al. Roentgenographic evaluation of lumbar spine flexion-extension in asymptomatic individuals. Spine 1989;14:327–31.

[19] Mimura M, Panjabi MM, Oxland TR, et al. Disc degeneration affects the multidirectional flexibility of the lumbar spine. Spine 1994;19:1371–80.

[20] Fujiwara A, Lim TH, An HS, et al. The effect of disc degeneration and facet joint osteoarthritis on the segmental flexibility of the lumbar spine. Spine 2000;25:3036–44.

[21] Coppes MH, Marani E, Thomeer RT, et al. Innervation of "painful" lumbar discs. Spine 1997;22:2342–9 [discussion: 9–50].

[22] Antonacci MD, Mody DR, Heggeness MH. Innervation of the human vertebral body: a histologic study. J Spinal Disord 1998;11:526–31.

[23] Brown MF, Hukkanen MV, McCarthy ID, et al. Sensory and sympathetic innervation of the vertebral endplate in patients with degenerative disc disease. J Bone Joint Surg Br 1997;79:147–53.

[24] Bertagnoli R, Kumar S. Indications for full prosthetic disc arthroplasty: a correlation of clinical outcome against a variety of indications. Eur Spine J 2002;11(Suppl 2):S131–6.

[25] Huang RC, Lim MR, Girardi FP, et al. The prevalence of contraindications to total disc replacement in a cohort of lumbar surgical patients. Spine 2004;29:2538–41.

[26] Weinhoffer SL, Guyer RD, Herbert M, et al. Intradiscal pressure measurements above an instrumented fusion. A cadaveric study. Spine 1995;20:526–31.

[27] Eck JC, Humphreys SC, Lim TH, et al. Biomechanical study on the effect of cervical spine fusion on adjacent level intradiscal pressure and segmental motion. Spine 2002;27:2431–4.

[28] Maiman DJ, Kumaresan S, Yoganandan N, et al. Biomechanical effect of anterior cervical spine fusion on adjacent segments. Biomed Mater Eng 1999;9:27–38.

[29] Goto K, Tajima N, Chosa E, et al. Effects of lumbar spinal fusion on the other lumbar intervertebral levels (three-dimensional finite element analysis). J Orthop Sci 2003;8:577–84.

[30] Phillips FM, Reuben J, Wetzel FT. Intervertebral disc degeneration adjacent to a lumbar fusion. An experimental rabbit model. J Bone Joint Surg Br 2002;84:289–94.

[31] Whitecloud III TS, Davis JM, Olive PM. Operative treatment of the degenerated segment adjacent to a lumbar fusion. Spine 1994;19:531–6.

[32] Lee CK. Accelerated degeneration of the segment adjacent to a lumbar fusion. Spine 1988;13:375–7.

[33] Ghiselli G, Wang JC, Bhatia NN, et al. Adjacent segment degeneration in the lumbar spine. J Bone Joint Surg Am 2004;86:1497–503.

[34] Hilibrand AS, Carlson GD, Palumbo MA, et al. Radiculopathy and myelopathy at segments adjacent to the site of a previous anterior cervical arthrodesis. J Bone Joint Surg Am 1999;81:519–28.

[35] Kumar MN, Baklanov A, Chopin D. Correlation between sagittal plane changes and adjacent segment degeneration following lumbar spine fusion. Eur Spine J 2001;10:314–9.

[36] Katsuura A, Hukuda S, Saruhashi Y, et al. Kyphotic malalignment after anterior cervical fusion is one of the factors promoting the degenerative process in adjacent intervertebral levels. Eur Spine J 2001;10:320–4.

[37] Akamaru T, Kawahara N, Tim Yoon S, et al. Adjacent segment motion after a simulated lumbar fusion in different sagittal alignments: a biomechanical analysis. Spine 2003;28:1560–6.

[38] Silva M, Shepherd EF, Jackson WO, et al. Average patient walking activity approaches 2 million cycles per year: pedometers under-record walking activity. J Arthroplasty 2002;17:693–7.

[39] Szpalski M, Gunzburg R, Mayer M. Spine arthroplasty: a historical review. Eur Spine J 2002;11(Suppl 2): S65–84.

[40] Cinotti G, David T, Postacchini F. Results of disc prosthesis after a minimum follow-up period of 2 years. Spine 1996;21:995–1000.

[41] Tropiano P, Huang RC, Girardi FP, et al. Clinical results of lumbar total disc replacement at 9-year follow-up. Hospital for Special Surgery 85th Alumni Association Meeting. New York, New York, 2003.

[42] Granberry WM, Noble PC, Bishop JO, et al. Use of a hinged silicone prosthesis for replacement arthroplasty of the first metatarsophalangeal joint. J Bone Joint Surg Am 1991;73:1453–9.

[43] Lundkvist L, Barfred T. Total wrist arthroplasty. Experience with Swanson flexible silicone implants, 1982–1988. Scand J Plast Reconstr Surg Hand Surg 1992;26:97–100.

[44] Freed JB. The increasing recognition of medullary lysis, cortical osteophytic proliferation, and fragmentation of implanted silicone polymer implants. J Foot Ankle Surg 1993;32:171–9.

[45] Trepman E, Ewald FC. Early failure of silicone radial head implants in the rheumatoid elbow. A complication of silicone radial head implant arthroplasty. J Arthroplasty 1991;6:59–65.

[46] Enker P, Steffee A, McMillin C, et al. Artificial disc replacement. Preliminary report with a 3-year minimum follow-up. Spine 1993;18:1061–70.

[47] Huang RC, Girardi FP, Cammisa Jr FP, et al. The implications of constraint in lumbar total disc replacement. J Spinal Disord Tech 2003;16:412–7.

[48] Zeegers WS, Bohnen LM, Laaper M, et al. Artificial disc replacement with the modular type SB Charite III: 2-year results in 50 prospectively studied patients. Eur Spine J 1999;8:210–7.

[49] Lemaire JP, Skalli W, Lavaste F, et al. Intervertebral disc prosthesis. Results and prospects for the year 2000. Clin Orthop 1997;337:64–76.

[50] Tropiano P, Huang RC, Girardi FP, et al. Lumbar disc replacement: preliminary results with ProDisc II after a minimum follow-up period of 1 year. J Spinal Disord Tech 2003;16:362–8.

[51] Bryan Jr VE. Cervical motion segment replacement. Eur Spine J 2002;11(Suppl 2):S92–7.

[52] Wigfield CC, Gill SS, Nelson RJ, et al. The new Frenchay artificial cervical joint: results from a two-year pilot study. Spine 2002;27:2446–52.

[53] Goffin J, Van Calenbergh F, Van Loon J, et al. Intermediate follow-up after treatment of degenerative disc disease with the Bryan Cervical Disc prosthesis: single-level and bi-level. Spine 2003;28:2673–8.

[54] Huang RC, Girardi FP, Cammisa Jr FP, et al. Long-term flexion-extension range of motion of the prodisc total disc replacement. J Spinal Disord Tech 2003;16: 435–40.

[55] Putzier M, Schneider SV, Disch AC, et al. Clinical and radiological results after artificial disc replacement: 17-year long term follow-up. Eurospine 2004: Annual Meeting of the Spine Society of Europe. Porto, Portugal, 2004.

[56] Huang RC, Girardi FP, Cammisa Jr FP, et al. The relationship between range of motion and outcome in lumbar total disc replacement at 9-year follow-up. The International Society for the Study of the Lumbar Spine 31st Annual Meeting. Porto, Portugal, 2004.

[57] Huang RC, Girardi FP, Lim MR, et al. Range of motion and adjacent level degeneration after lumbar total disc replacement. Scoliosis Research Society 39th Annual Meeting. Buenos Aires, Argentina, 2004.

[58] Dooris AP, Goel VK, Grosland NM, et al. Load-sharing between anterior and posterior elements in a lumbar motion segment implanted with an artificial disc. Spine 2001;26:E122–9.

[59] Steffen T, Tsantrizos A, Aebi M. Effect of implant design and endplate preparation on the compressive strength of interbody fusion constructs. Spine 2000; 25:1077–84.

[60] Grant JP, Oxland TR, Dvorak MF. Mapping the structural properties of the lumbosacral vertebral endplates. Spine 2001;26:889–96.

[61] Panjabi MM, Chen NC, Shin EK, et al. The cortical shell architecture of human cervical vertebral bodies. Spine 2001;26:2478–84.

[62] Klara PM, Ray CD. Artificial nucleus replacement: clinical experience. Spine 2002;27:1374–7.

[63] Bertagnoli R, Schonmayr R. Surgical and clinical results with the PDN prosthetic disc-nucleus device. Eur Spine J 2002;11(Suppl 2):S143–8.

[64] Mulholland RC, Sengupta DK. Rationale, principles and experimental evaluation of the concept of soft stabilization. Eur Spine J 2002;11(Suppl 2):S198–205.

[65] Sengupta DK. Dynamic stabilization devices in the treatment of low back pain. Orthop Clin North Am 2004;35:43–56.

[66] Graf H. Lumbar instability: surgical treatment without fusion. Rachis 1992;412:123–37.
[67] Hadlow SV, Fagan AB, Hillier TM, Fraser RD. The Graf ligamentoplasty procedure. Comparison with posterolateral fusion in the management of low back pain. Spine 1998;23:1172–9.
[68] Brechbuhler D, Markwalder TM, Braun M. Surgical results after soft system stabilization of the lumbar spine in degenerative disc disease–long-term results. Acta Neurochir (Wien) 1998;140:521–5.
[69] Grevitt MP, Gardner AD, Spilsbury J, et al. The Graf stabilisation system: early results in 50 patients. Eur Spine J 1995;4:169–75 [discussion: 35].
[70] Madan S, Boeree NR. Outcome of the Graf ligamentoplasty procedure compared with anterior lumbar interbody fusion with the Hartshill horseshoe cage. Eur Spine J 2003;12:361–8.
[71] Konno S, Kikuchi S. Prospective study of surgical treatment of degenerative spondylolisthesis: comparison between decompression alone and decompression with graf system stabilization. Spine 2000;25:1533–7.
[72] Hashimoto T, Oha F, Shigenobu K, et al. Mid-term clinical results of Graf stabilization for lumbar degenerative pathologies. A minimum 2-year follow-up. Spine J 2001;1:283–9.
[73] Stoll TM, Dubois G, Schwarzenbach O. The dynamic neutralization system for the spine: a multi-center study of a novel non-fusion system. Eur Spine J 2002; 11(Suppl 2):S170–8.
[74] Schmoelz W, Huber JF, Nydegger T, et al. Dynamic stabilization of the lumbar spine and its effects on adjacent segments: an in vitro experiment. J Spinal Disord Tech 2003;16:418–23.

Standard and Minimally Invasive Approaches to the Spine

Ronald A. Lehman, Jr, MD[a], Alexander R. Vaccaro, MD[b,*], Rudolf Bertagnoli, MD[c], Timothy R. Kuklo, MD[a]

[a]*Department of Orthopaedic Surgery, Walter Reed Army Medical Center, Washington DC 20307, USA*
[b]*Department of Orthopedic Surgery, Thomas Jefferson University and the Rothman Institute, Philadelphia, PA 19107, USA*
[c]*Spine Center, St.-Elisabeth-Klinikum, St.-Elisabeth-Str. 23, 94315 Straubing, Germany*

With the advent of minimally invasive surgical approaches to the spine, the ability to adequately expose the desired anatomic structures while minimizing the disadvantages of excessive soft tissue stripping, dissection, and prolonged retraction has become increasingly popular. For example, the traditional posterior surgical approach to the lumbar spine involves making a midline longitudinal incision of sufficient length to expose the desired spinal levels, stripping the paraspinal muscles from the posterior spinal elements, and statically retracting the superficial and deep paraspinal muscles to allow for adequate visualization and hemostasis throughout the surgical procedure. Several studies have demonstrated that prolonged soft tissue retraction generates a greater force per unit area on the retracted soft tissues, resulting in an increase in the degree of regional ischemia, leading to paraspinal electromyogram abnormalities and decreased muscle density. Muscle weakness and denervation are critical consequences resulting in potentially long-term adverse side effects such as chronic pain and muscular dysfunction. The surgeons' ability to minimize soft tissue dissection translates into less acute postoperative pain, necessitates less narcotic pain medication, and often shortens hospital stays.

One of the drawbacks to minimally invasive surgery entails the lengthy learning curve necessary to master the various techniques. The difficulty of positioning instrumentation and implants in a confined space and the acuity of using two-dimensional aids to infer depth perception often adds significant time to the procedure. The most popular minimal-access spinal procedures have been used in posterior cervical and lumbar procedures and thoracoscopy for herniated thoracic discs or ligament release. Laparoscopic transperitoneal or balloon-assisted retroperitoneal anterior lumbar procedures have fallen out of favor due to the equivalency of effectiveness and improved safety of miniopen techniques.

Minimal-access procedures often rely on the development of a surgical corridor through the placement of sequential dilators or a retraction tube over the desired anatomic location. Tube visualization has now graduated to independent retractable blades, allowing multisegment visualization. This methodology has proved to be simpler than increasing the diameter of a fixed circular retractor and easier in terms of freedom of instrument manipulation and implant delivery than that afforded with distally expandable retractors with a fixed proximal aperture. Using an endoscopic light source or external focused lighting such as a microscope or headlight, more contemporary minimal-access approaches allow for direct visualization of spinal anatomy, thus avoiding reliance on indirect visualization using an endoscopic monitor.

The opinions or assertions contained herein are the private views of the authors and are not to be construed as official or as reflecting the views of the United States Army or the Department of Defense.

* Corresponding author.

E-mail address: alexvaccaro3@aol.com (A.R. Vaccaro).

Cervical approaches

Posterior approach to the cervical spine

The midline open approach to the posterior cervical spine is the most commonly used approach to access the posterior cervical elements because it allows for safe and reproducible exposure of the posterior cervical spine for a myriad of indications (Fig. 1) [1]. In a patient without a previous posterior decompressive procedure, an open exposure of the posterior cervical spine is relatively straightforward [2–8]. Dissection along the midline between the paraspinal muscles within the central raphe minimizes bleeding and iatrogenic muscle trauma.

Positioning
The patient is placed prone on the table, with the neck flexed slightly to facilitate opening of the interspinous spaces and held in place with a Mayfield headrest (Integra, Neurosciences, Plainsboro, New Jersey) or other rigid headrest. The table is manipulated into the reverse Trendelenburg position to align the cervical spine horizontally and aid fluid drainage away from the surgical field. This position also allows for compression or collapse of the epidural vessels, thereby decreasing the risk of air emboli.

Landmarks and anatomy
The C2, C7, and T1 spinous processes are among the most prominent landmarks in the posterior cervical spine and are easily palpable even in larger individuals. There is often difficulty in differentiating C7 from T1; therefore, a spinal needle may be placed and a lateral radiograph obtained to determine the proper level. In addition, C7 is thicker and not usually bifid like the cephalad vertebral levels and has a tubercle at its end.

Incision and dissection
A straight midline incision is made centered over the spinous processes of interest. Surgeons should be aware that the skin over the posterior cervical spine is much thicker than the skin along the anterior aspect of the neck. The internervous plane is between the left and right paracervical muscles, which are segmentally innervated by the left and right posterior rami of the cervical nerves.

At the level of the lamina, the paraspinal muscles may be elevated subperiosteally with a Cobb spinal elevator (Apothecaries Sundries Mfg. Co., New Delhi, India). A bilateral exposure is frequently necessary for fusion, whereas a unilateral approach is used for a foraminotomy. The dissection can be carried as far laterally as needed to visualize the lamina, facet joints, and the lateral masses. The segmental arteries may need to be cauterized because the posterior cervical musculature is vascular.

Posterior minimally invasive approach to the cervical spine

Lateral fluoroscopy or plain radiography is used to identify the desired surgical level. The starting point is approximately 2 to 3 cm lateral to the midline. Anteroposterior fluoroscopy assists in determining the starting position in the transverse plane. A guide wire or preferably a blunt cannula is navigated with use of orthogonal imaging to rest on the cephalad lamina of the facet joint of interest. Following this, a 2-cm incision is made about the Kirschner wire (RFQ-Medizintechnik GmbH & Co. KG, Tuttlingen, Germany) or blunt cannula, and then sequential dilators are used to expand the soft tissue to mature a corridor down to the posterior spinal elements. The dilator may be used to dissect the soft tissue from the lamina above and below the desired level (Fig. 2). On the outside of the dilator, a measuring scale facilitates blade length choice for the final expandable retractor. The expandable dilator is now placed and manipulated to facilitate visualization of the surgical level. A light source can be connected to the dilator system, and assisted visualization is afforded by way of a microscope or loupe magnification and possibly a headlight. This technique is excellent for single- or two-level foraminotomies and provides significant

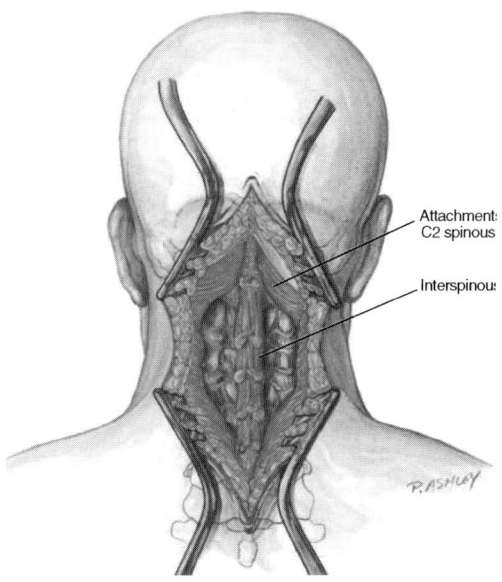

Fig. 1. Posterior cervical spine exposure.

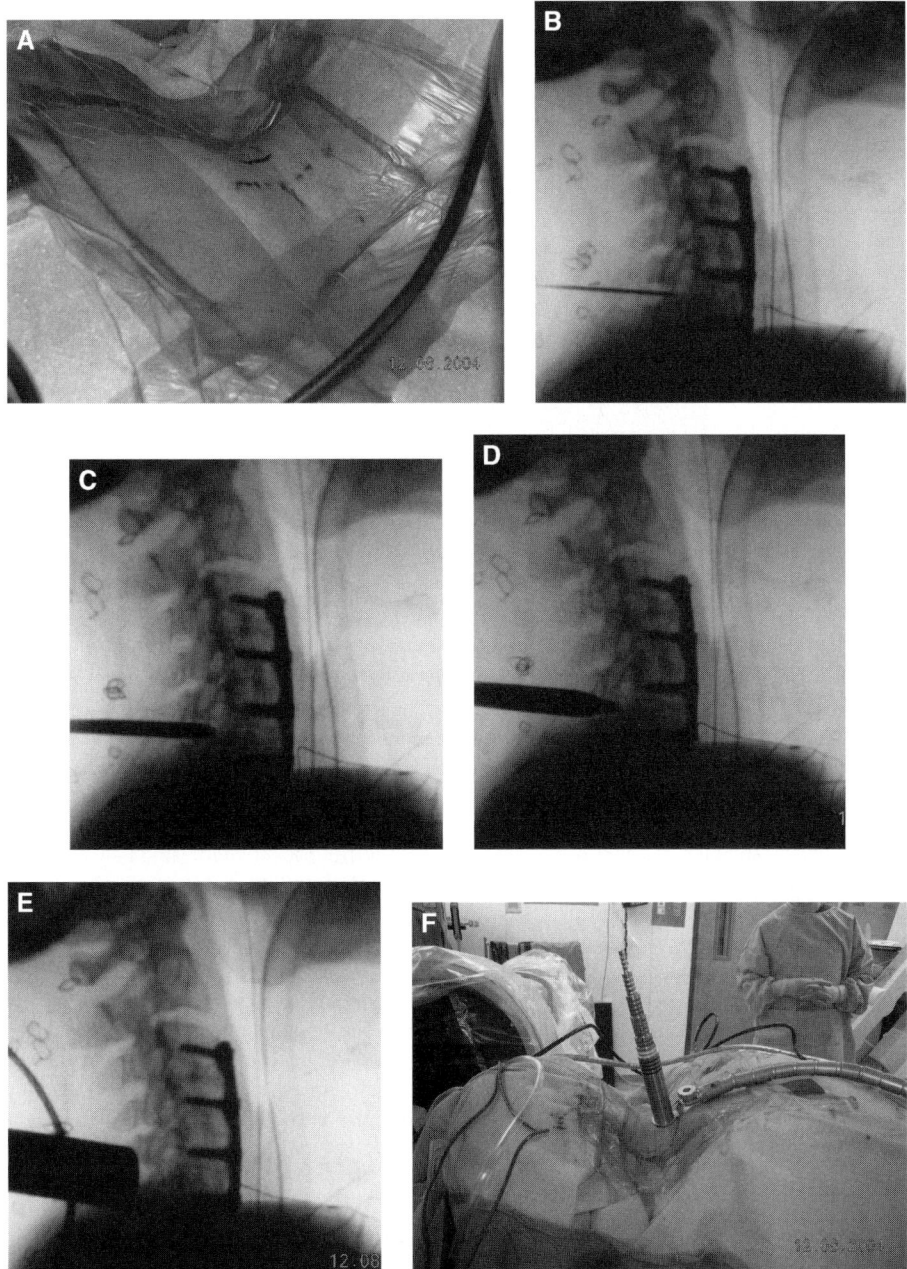

Fig. 2. Thirty-seven-year-old man with posterior foraminal impingement and left C6 radiculopathy secondary to bony foraminal disc after successful three-level anterior cervical diskectomy and fusion. (*A*) Patient positioning with skin marker over incision site, approximately 3 cm lateral to the midline. (*B–E*) Sequential insertion of guide wire and dilating tubes. (*F*) Placement of endoscopic tube and connector. (*G*) Microscopic view of posterior interlaminar space through tube. (*H*) After extended forminotomy and bony disc removal, with arrows on spinal cord and exiting C6 nerve root. (*I*) Closure of skin incision.

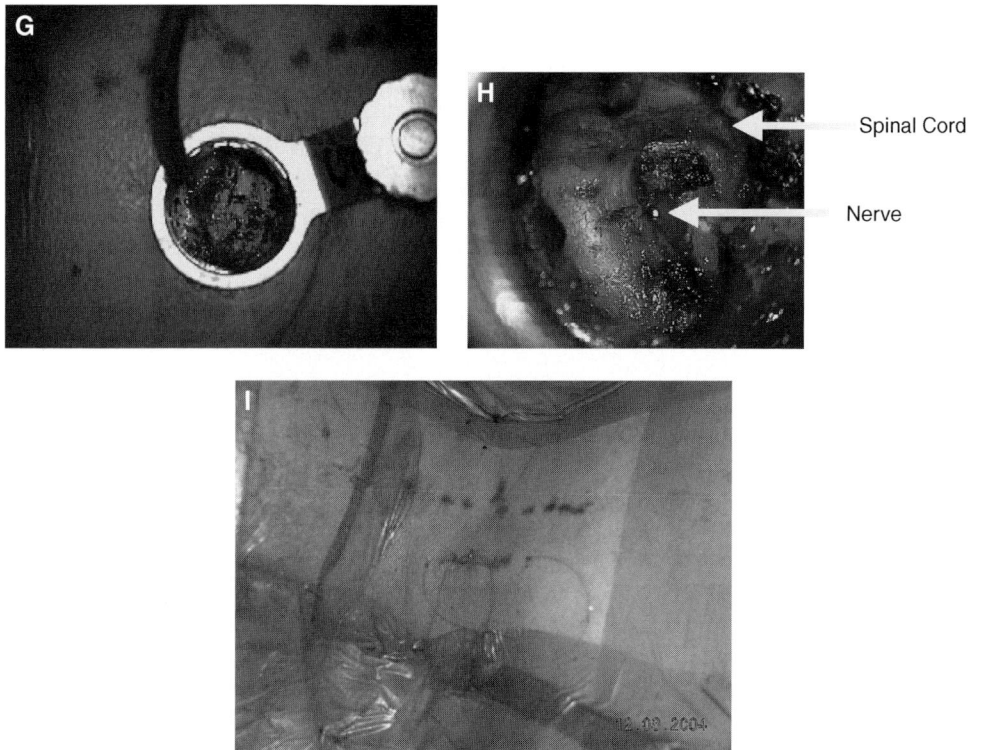

Fig. 2 (*continued*).

postoperative reduction in pain secondary to the decreased muscle retraction and avoidance of subperiosteal stripping.

An example of an expandable retractor is the MAXCESS minimally invasion decompressive system and instruments (NuVasive, San Diego, California). This device uses a split radiolucent blade design that allows for use in conventional and minimally invasive procedures. Cranial, caudal, and medial or lateral independently controlled retractors allow for ease of exposure of the spinal elements.

Anterior approach to the cervical spine

The most commonly used standard approach to the anterior cervical spine is the Smith-Robinson approach. It is generally considered for exposure to the subaxial spine (ie, from C3 through T1) but has also been described with extension to the upper cervical spine [9]. This approach is performed on both sides, depending on surgeon preference. For instance, right-handed surgeons may prefer a right-sided approach, whereas others prefer a left-sided approach due to the more aberrant course of the right recurrent laryngeal nerve as it crosses the field around C5-6 after hooking around the right subclavian artery and running alongside the trachea in the neck [10]. Dissection proceeds medial to the anterior border of the sternocleidomastoid muscle and deeper between the carotid sheath laterally and the trachea and esophagus medially. Care must be taken to avoid the hypoglossal, glossop, and superior laryngeal nerves, especially because the dissection is carried cephalad. Specifically, injury to the superior laryngeal nerve may result in dysphagia, voice changes, and an inability to phonate high notes [2,11,12]. The carotid sheath, which contains the internal jugular vein, the common carotid artery, and the vagus nerve, lies under the sternocleidomastoid muscle and is retracted laterally. All of these structures are usually protected with meticulous blunt dissection and careful retraction. The use of intraoperative electrodiagnostic techniques has been recommended to avoid injury to the facial nerve; however, this method of surveillance is not widely accepted by spinal surgeons.

The patient is placed supine on the operating room table, with the head and neck rotated slightly away from the intended operative side. The endotracheal tube is also taped opposite from the operative field. A soft roll is placed under the scapulae to provide slight extension of the cervical spine. The table should be placed in reverse Trendelenburg to reduce venous bleeding during the procedure.

The application of a distractive force may be appropriate, especially when performing an interbody fusion or multilevel surgery. Skeleton traction may be applied with the use of Gardner-Wells tongs (Jarit Instruments, Hawthorne, NY) with weights up to 10 to 15 lb. This technique is beneficial because it can be used to provide continuous traction and stability to the spine, especially after a multilevel corpectomy or trauma. Also, head halter traction may be used, which obviates the need for skeletal traction. Care must be taken to avoid excessive traction to the brachial plexus with this method if concomitant downward traction through taping is employed to the shoulders.

After the skin is incised, the superficial fascia anterior to the platysma is gently elevated off the muscle. The platysma muscle is then divided longitudinally in line with its fibers, and flaps are developed superiorly and inferiorly. Next, the interval between the strap muscles and the anterior border of the sternocleidomastoid muscle must be identified and the fascia lying anterior to the muscle incised. This procedure can be done with gentle finger dissection or with the use of surgical instruments. Dissection in a cranial and a caudal direction at each level significantly enhances visualization when using a transverse skin incision.

Following incision of the cervical fascia over the medial border of the sternocleidomastoid muscle, the pretracheal fascia is identified and dissected medial to the carotid sheath. Palpation of the carotid artery aids in the identification of the carotid sheath and its contents. The dissection should proceed medial to the carotid sheath and lateral to the esophagus and trachea. This procedure may be performed with blunt dissection and palpation or direct visualization. After palpation of the cartotid artery, it is gently retracted laterally to remove it from the operative field. The superior and inferior thyroid arteries, which connect the carotid sheath with the midline structures, may limit the superior dissection. These vessels are typically noted superficial to the cervical vertebrae and may be ligated to enhance exposure. The retropharyngeal space is then entered over the anterior aspect of the vertebral bodies. The cervical vertebrae can now be visualized along with the longus colli muscles bilaterally and the prevertebral fascia. In addition, the anterior longitudinal ligament can be seen in the midline as a gleaming white structure. The sympathetic chain lies on the longus colli, just lateral to the vertebral bodies. It is important to discern between the alar fascia (superficial to the prevertebral fascia), which invests the carotid sheath, and the visceral fascia, which envelops the esophagus and the recurrent laryngeal nerve. The plane between the alar and visceral fascia should be developed to widen the exposure. With the use of electrocautery or Cobb elevators, the longus colli is split longitudinally over the midline of the vertebral bodies. The medial edge of the muscle should be subperiosteally dissected with electrocautery along with the anterior longitudinal ligament. The disc spaces ("hills") can be differentiated from the vertebral bodies ("valleys"). It is important to ensure that the cervical retractors are placed deep to the longus colli muscles as they are opened. This methodology allows optimal visualization of the anterior cervical spinal elements and protects the recurrent laryngeal nerve, trachea, and esophagus. After the retractors are maximally opened, the endotracheal cuff may be deflated and reinflated to centralize the cuff and, theoretically, minimize pressure on internal branches of the recurrent laryngeal nerve within the endolarynx. A spinal needle can be placed within the disc space while a lateral radiograph is obtained to identify the surgical level.

Anterior minimally invasive approach to the cervical spine

A similar series of sequences is repeated for minimal-access procedures to expose the anterior cervical spine. The surgeon exploits similar dissection planes using techniques and instruments similar to an open procedure but through a skin aperture of approximately 2 cm. After the spine is reached, visualization is performed through an expandable or nonexpandable cannula system.

Thoracic and thoracolumbar approaches

Anterior thoracolumbar extensile approach

The anterior thoracolumbar extensile approach is used to gain access to the distal thoracic and proximal lumbar spine. This extensile approach provides excellent visualization of the anterior spinal column and can be performed from either side. Because the major arterial vessels lie on the left side, however, some investigators advocate approaching from the left to mobilize the vessels more easily. Often, the side of the pathology or the location of the curve convexity in spinal deformity dictates the side of the approach. This approach can be extended from the upper thoracic to the lower lumbar spine.

The patient is placed in the lateral decubitus position with the use of a beanbag positioning device. It is important that a double-lumen endotracheal tube be used for single lung ventilation during the procedure. The incision can be made anywhere along the ninth through eleventh rib. The skin incision is made over the rib, beginning posteriorly and extending anteriorly and distally to the level of the symphysis pubis if necessary. The latissimus dorsi muscle is split along with the serratus anterior, thereby exposing the desired rib. The rib is subsequently removed in a subperiosteal manner and may be used as bone graft. It is imperative to make the incision in the cephalad half of the rib to avoid compromise of the neurovascular bundle that lies on the inferior posterior margin of the rib. After removal of the rib, the pleural cavity is opened through the periosteal rib bed and the retroperitoneal space is entered. The peritoneum is visualized and dissected off the deep abdominal muscles bluntly from anterior lateral to posterior medial. After reflection of the peritoneum, the internal oblique and transversus abdominus muscles are incised as needed. Next, the peritoneum is bluntly swept off the psoas muscle from the undersurface of the diaphragm, thereby exposing the retroperitoneal space. The diaphragm is incised circumferentially, leaving a 1-cm cuff to aid in future repair. After the spine is visualized, the segmental vessels are identified and ligated as necessary. It is important to ligate these vessels approximately 1 cm from the intervertebral foramen to allow for collateral circulation. At this point, adequate exposure of the thoracolumbar spine can be appreciated and the pathology addressed as indicated. Following the procedure, a chest tub is placed, the diaphragm is repaired, the rib bed closed, and the lung reinflated.

Anterior miniopen retroperitoneal approach to the lower lumbar spine

The anterior miniopen retroperitoneal approach to the lower lumbar spine [13,14] is often performed with the patient positioned supine on the operating room table. The patient is placed in a slight Trendelenburg position and rolled toward the right to allow the visceral contents to fall with gravity away from the side of the approach. The surgeon confirms the disc space or vertebral levels to be approached on a lateral fluoroscopic view. If a two-level procedure is performed, then the incision is made slightly inferior to the midpoint between the two levels. Some investigators prefer a vertical incision, whereas others recommend a horizontal incision for cosmetic reasons. The surgeon typically stands on the right side of the patient and works toward him- or herself. For an L5-S1 exposure, a 4-cm transverse skin incision is made 1 cm to the right of the midline that extends 3 cm to the left of the midline. The incision is located two- to three-finger breadths above the pubic symphysis. After sharp dissection through the skin and soft tissue, the rectus abdominus is encountered. The midline between the heads of the rectus is identified and bluntly dissected inferior to the arcuate line to allow entry into the retroperitoneal space. As this blunt dissection is carried distally, the retroperitoneal space is encountered and retracted from left to right. With the ureter and the peritoneum retracted, blunt dissection is continued until the sacral promontory is encountered. For complete exposure of the L5-S1 disc space, the left common iliac vein and middle sacral vessels are mobilized. The presacral plexus should be swept from the midline with blunt dissection. The middle sacral artery and vein are often adherent to the anterior anulus and may require ligation. After the disc is visualized and the proper level is confirmed radiographically, the disc may be removed. This technique is referred to as the miniopen approach because the initial skin incision may be as small as 4 cm. Tubular retractors (expandable) may be used to widen the exposure or the surgeon may select standard table-based retractor blades to assist in skin and soft tissue retraction (Fig. 3).

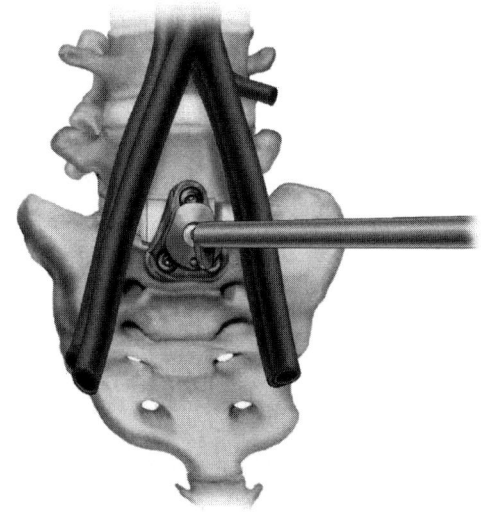

Fig. 3. Minimally invasive placement of anterior plate. (*Courtesy of* Medtronic Sofamor Danek, Memphis, Tennessee; with permission.)

Exposure of the L4-5 level is often more difficult because the great vessels bifurcate at that level. Typically, all of the major vessels are retracted to the right and exposure is obtained by proceeding posteriorly behind the vessels. If there is an alteration in the bifurcation level, the surgeon must adjust accordingly. Occasionally, the surgeon may mobilize the left common iliac artery and vein across the disc space. Often, the iliolumbar vein or the segmental vessels may need to be divided. The iliolumbar vein, if encountered, must be handled with caution because significant bleeding may occur with vessel disruption.

Anterolateral transpsoatic approach

To minimize the risk to the great vessels and viscus associated with the posterior approach, the anterolateral transpsoatic approach to L1 through L4 was developed [15]. This approach is ideal for use with an expandable retractor system after access is developed down to the level of the psoas muscle. The nucleus-replacing devices have typically been inserted through a posterior approach. Although this procedure has had success, there are still some major limitations/concerns with this approach; namely, damage to the facets with ligament and bone removal, dural exposure and excessive retraction on the nerve roots with possible epidural bleeding, and excessive scarring. Instead of approaching the spine anteriorly or anterolaterally, the disc is accessed laterally through the psoas muscle. A potential drawback of this exposure is the risk of injury to the femoral or genitofemoral nerves, although this complication has been reported to be transient. Moreover, because a large section of the disc can be exposed through this approach, placement and visualization of the implant is facilitated.

Positioning

Unlike the anterior approach to the lumbar spine whereby the patient is positioned supine, the anterolateral transpsoatic approach requires that the patient be positioned in a 90° lateral decubitus position on an adjustable table. Before the lateral incision is made, the exact location of intended exposure is identified and marked with the use of fluoroscopy.

The surgeon stands behind the patient before making the skin incision. A 2-cm vertical or transverse incision is made over the desired disc space and dissection proceeds in line with the fibers of the external oblique muscle. Blunt dissection is used to traverse the external and internal obliques, and the transverses muscles in the direction of their fibers. The retroperitoneal space is identified and protected medially along the lateral aspect of the psoas muscle. The disc is now accessed by way of blunt dissection through the psoas muscle fibers in contrast to the standard anterior approach whereby the spine is accessed anterior to the psoas muscle. The anatomic "safe-zone" is between the anterior third and posterior two thirds of the psoas muscle through a 2- to 3-cm window. This safe zone correlates with the lateral and middle third of the disc space. Care must be taken to avoid anterior surgical deviation by which injury to major blood vessels and the sympathetic chain may occur.

Balloon-assisted endoscopic retroperitoneal gasless technique

Another option for limiting the surgical incision during a lumbar procedure involves the use of the balloon-assisted endoscopic retroperitoneal gasless approach anteriorly [16]. This technique uses an inflatable balloon to widen the retroperitoneal space for ease of instrument and implant insertion. It avoids the need for gas insufflation, which was an older but popular minimally invasive means of exposure to L5-S1 and, in some cases, L4-5. The balloon-assisted endoscopic retroperitoneal gasless technique has fallen out of favor for the simpler and reproducible miniopen approach to the anterior lumbar spine.

Posterior approach to the lumbar spine

The posterior approach to the lumbar spine [13] begins with placement of the patient in the prone position on the operating room table. Before the surgical incision, the level of approach may be confirmed with anteroposterior and lateral plain radiographs or fluoroscopy. The patient must be properly padded so that the abdomen is able to hang freely. This position allows the nonvalvular vertebral venous plexus to empty freely into the vena cava, thereby reducing operative bleeding. A midline incision is made directed over the intended spinal levels. After incising the skin and subcutaneous tissue, the posterior paraspinal muscles are encountered. The posterior muscles of the thoracic and lumbar region are arranged in three layers: superficial, intermediate, and deep. These distinct layers are not visualized during the dissection but are retracted laterally as a collective group. Because of the muscular attachments on the lateral aspects of the spinous processes (especially in the thoracic region), careful adherence to midline dissection is prudent to avoid unnecessary bleeding. The rotator muscles pass in a lateral to medial direction, with the distal end of the muscle being more lateral. The resulting angle between the muscle and its insertion makes stripping the muscles in a caudad to cephalad direction in the thoracic region easier. The transverse processes should be stripped off in a distal to proximal direction as the transverse processes become larger from T12 to T1. Dissection should proceed cautiously to avoid injury to the posterior rami, which lie between the transverse processes lateral to the pars interarticularis and the facets and their capsules.

Wiltse approach

The original description of the paraspinal posterior approach to the lumbar spine was for spinal fusion, especially regarding lumbosacral spondylolisthesis treatment. The transmuscular paraspinal approach [17,18] takes into account the level of the natural cleavage plane between the multifidus and the longissimus part of the sacrospinalis muscle from the midline at the level of the spinous process of L4. A natural cleavage plane between the multifidus and the longissimus part of the sacrospinalis muscle is encountered, with a fibrous separation between the two muscles. The mean distance between the level of the cleavage plane and the midline is approximately 4 cm. In all cases, small arteries and veins are present at the level of the cleavage plane. After encountering the cleavage plane, it is easy to localize it between the multifidus and the longissimus part of the sacrospinalis muscle. First, the superficial muscular fascia is opened near the midline, exposing the posterior aspect of the sacrospinalis muscle. The location of the muscular cleft can then be found by identifying the perforating vessels, leaving the anatomic intermuscular space. This dissection is carried down to the level of the desired vertebral level.

Placement of posterior segmental spinal instrumentation

The greatest challenge to the spine surgeon is the placement of segmental spinal fixation (pedicle screws or lateral mass screws) in a minimally invasive manner [19–25]. There are several popular techniques in use today to accomplish this task. One involves the use of a distally expansive tube retractor system relying on the use of an attached fiber-optic light source, microscope, or endoscopic two-dimensional visualization of implant site application and fluoroscopic imaging to guide implant trajectory. Another method uses orthogonal fluoroscopic or computer image guidance to percutaneously place guide wires within the pedicle that ultimately guide screw placement. The placement of the longitudinal connector (rod) with this method is guided by an attached spinal anchor frame that directs the rod into the spinal anchors. Possibly the easiest technique is the recent introduction of expandable tube retractors that are placed through a small incision and allow direct visualization of implant starting points, with screw path trajectory aided by the use of lateral fluoroscopy.

The use of an adjustable or expandable retractor allows the surgeon to exploit familiar surgical skills to access the spine through a smaller incision, which may be widened through retractor expansion without lengthening the skin incision [20]. A myriad of surgical procedures can now be readily performed with this method using direct visualization, avoiding the two-dimensional sight constraints of spinal endoscopy. Common procedures suitable for this approach include decompressive laminectomies, foraminotomies, discectomies, posterolateral and interbody fusions, and multilevel (two motion segment) pedicle screw placement whereby the tube can expand on independent blades along its length (Fig. 4). These systems allow the surgeon to visualize two to three spinal anchor starting points directly, similar to an open spinal procedure. These systems can be tailored to individual patient girth by exchanging or modifying the individual blades with in situ extension shims to address variations in local anatomy. The independent-blade design allows operative instruments to be leveraged against the incision border through openings between the blades during retractor expansion (Fig. 5). A multisegmented fusion can easily be performed without the need for

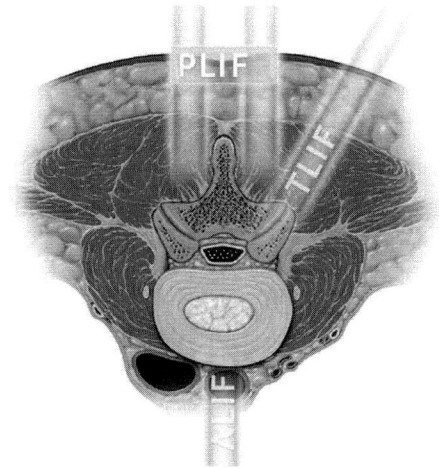

Fig. 4. Schematic depicting anterior lumbar interbody fusion (ALIF), posterior lumbar interbody fusion (PLIF), and transforaminal lumbar interbody fusion (TLIF) percutanous approaches. (*Courtesy of* Medtronic Sofamor Danek, Memphis, Tennessee; with permission.)

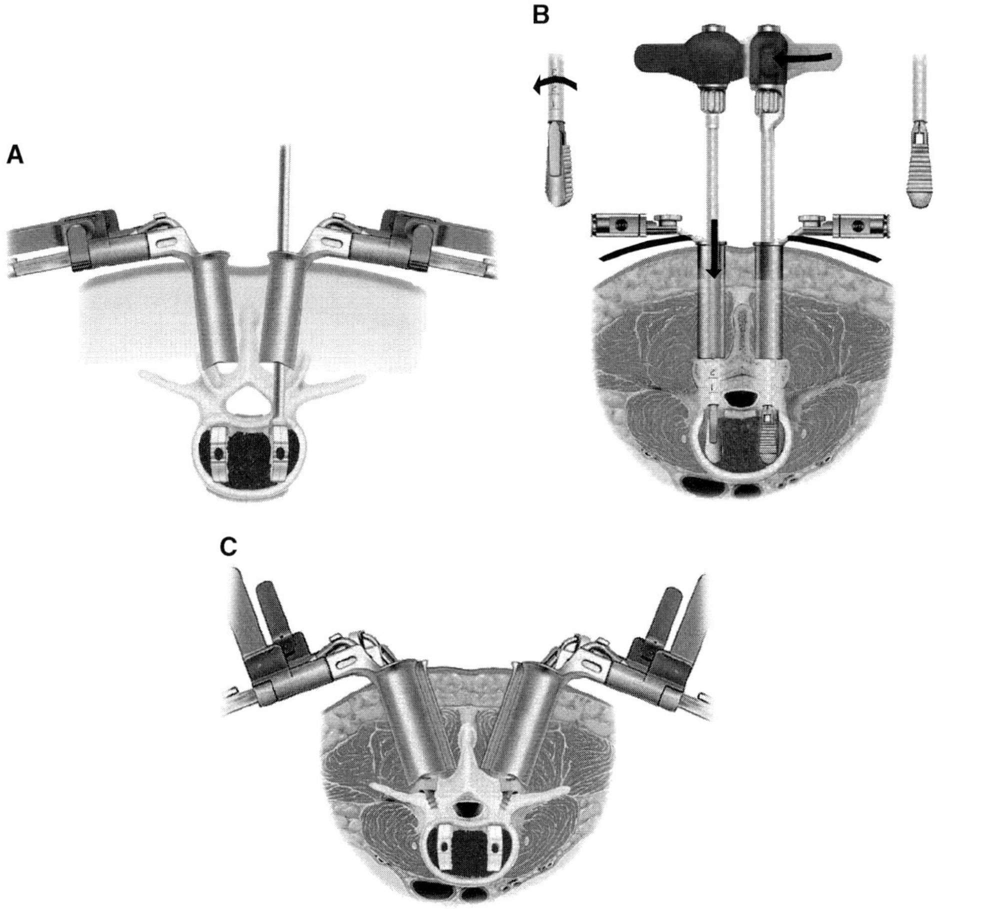

Fig. 5. (*A–C*). Axial schematics of posterior minimally invasive techniques. (*Courtesy of* Medtronic Sofamor Danek, Memphis, Tennessee; with permission.)

biplanar fluoroscopy or adjunctive guidance systems for rod delivery (Fig. 6). Lateral fluoroscopy or plain radiographs are recommended to confirm sagittal-plane screw trajectory.

Operative technique
Preparation and positioning. The patient is placed in the standard prone position on a radiolucent table such as a Jackson table (Orthopedic Systems, Inc., Hayword, CA). A bedrail should be present on the table to allow attachment of an articulating arm that stabilizes the retractor system after being inserted into the spinal incision.

Exposure. Fluoroscopy in the lateral (adequate) or anteroposterior and lateral planes is used to locate the desired spinal level or segment. The spinous process is palpated to define the midline. At the level of the

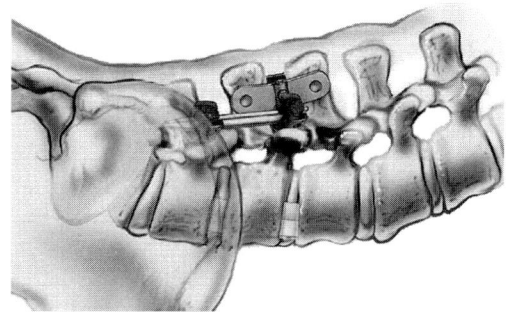

Fig. 6. Depiction after completion of interbody support and posterior rod screw construct placement. (*Courtesy of* Medtronic Sofamor Danek, Memphis, Tennessee; with permission.)

desired disc space, an incision point is marked on the skin approximately 3 to 4 cm lateral from the midline. A spinal needle or blunt trochar is introduced into the skin using fluoroscopic guidance to verify the desired spinal docking site. A 2- to 3-cm longitudinal incision is made at the site of the spinal needle or trochar entry point, and blunt dissection is taken down through the level of the superficial and deep fascia to easily accommodate subsequent spinal dilators. The path created by the trochar can be widened by the surgeon's fingers by removing the needle or trochar to initially widen the surgical path. The trochar is then replaced and advanced carefully through the superficial and deep fascia, making sure to not advance through the interlaminar space. Next, successively increasing dilating tubes are inserted with intermittent fluoroscopy to verify their position (Fig. 7). The depth of the last dilator is noted

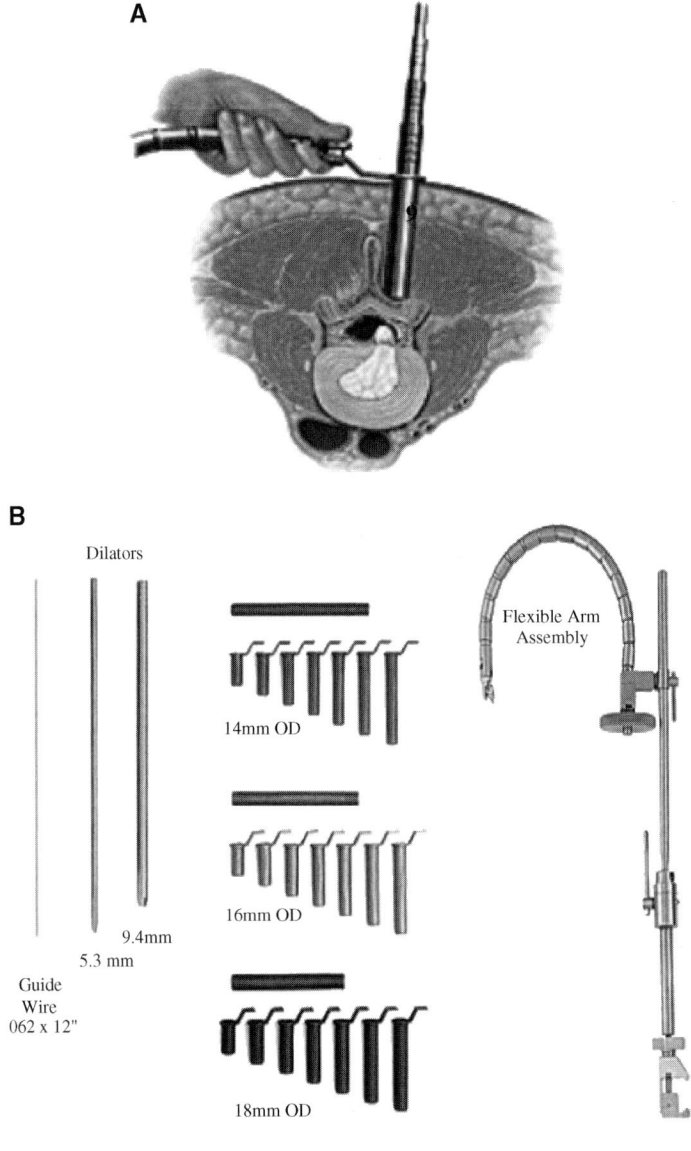

Fig. 7. (*A*) METRx Tube Retractor System (Medtronic Sofamor Danek). (*B*) Dilating tube system depicting tube sizes and flexible arm assembly. (*Courtesy of* Medtronic Sofamor Danek, Memphis, Tennessee; with permission.)

and the corresponding retractor blades are attached. The device is directed down to the facet joint and must be slanted obliquely toward the midline to guarantee adequate exposure. The articulating arm is attached to the contralateral bedrail and locked in place.

Complications

Only recently has minimally invasive spinal access become commonplace in posterior lumbar degenerative spinal procedures. Therefore, published data regarding complications represent only preliminary results. Long-term follow-up is required to determine the relative risks and benefits of minimal-access surgery compared with more traditional open procedures. Complications related to the surgical exposure are rare. The major difficulty with minimal-access procedures is the lack of adequate visualization for safe and reproducible neural decompression and implant placement. Systems that rely on indirect biplanar fluoroscopy for guide wire placement risk the potential for pedicle violation and implant canal intrusion with eccentric wire placement within the pedicle boundaries. Lack of clear, direct visualization of the neural elements risks the potential for dural violation or stretch neuropraxia.

Minimal access para-midline exposures require significantly less soft tissue dissection and, therefore, morbidity due to the blunt muscle-splitting approach compared with the requisite soft tissue stripping associated with an open midline procedure. Risks more pronounced with minimal-access surgery are primarily related to visualization. Specific complications such as a dural tear are much more difficult to repair using a minimal-access exposure. The advantage of a minimal-access approach that avoids the need for biplanar fluoroscopy or endoscopy is that it mimics the surgical skills used in open procedures and thus avoids the prolonged learning curve associated with traditional minimally invasive spinal procedures.

Summary

Over the last several years, minimal-access exposure of the posterior spine has become more popular as newer access tools have been developed and refined, minimizing the morbidity and shortening the learning curve of previous endoscopic techniques. It has also become a popular choice for patients educated in the morbidities related to extensive soft tissue dissection and retraction commonly associated with open spinal procedures. The minimization of soft tissue dissection, the reduction of local paraspinal muscle tension and ischemia, and the reduction of intraoperative blood loss associated with minimal-access surgery have led to shorter hospital stays and a more accelerated recovery time. The early experience with expandable-blade retractor systems for minimal-access decompression has been extremely encouraging. These systems are easily adjustable for customized exposure and provide superior illumination and visibility, affording the ability to perform multisegmental pedicle screw fixation through an open, direct surgical exposure, similar to open conventional procedures. The improved longitudinal and medial-lateral visibility offered by an independent blade retractor system appears to have significantly alleviated the access-related limitations experienced with static tubular systems or fluoroscopy-dependent implant-guided systems.

The percutaneous spinal systems have demonstrated great success as a minimally invasive procedure for pedicle screw/rod placement; however, if the length of the three parallel incisions required for the placement of two ipsilateral screws and the introduction of the longitudinal connector (rod) percutaneously is measured, it is often comparable to or even greater than the single 2-in incision needed for successful use of an expandable-blade access system and paramedian fixation construct placement. In addition to the need for healing of three separate ipsilateral incisions, greater muscular disruption is required for rod placement with these systems due to the long-swing arm of the rod compared with the single, smaller muscle-splitting, direct Wiltse-type approach provided by expandable tube systems.

A minimally invasive one- or two-level posterior exposure of the spine is now safely attainable with the latest minimal-access systems that exploit the biomechanics of an adjustable blade retractor. This technique is proving to be a valuable alternative operative approach to traditional open procedures. As the clinical use of these developing systems escalates, more outcomes data will become available to determine the value of these minimally invasive procedures.

Acceptance of minimal-access approaches will be slower in spinal surgery than other surgical specialties due to the risks of neural injury in cases of misadventure. A slow conversion to minimal-access approaches will generally mimic modifications of traditional open approaches until safety records can be established and reproduced.

References

[1] Rogers WA. Fractures and dislocations of the cervical spine; an end-result study. J Bone Joint Surg [Am] 1987;39:341–76.

[2] Epstein JA. The surgical management of cervical canal stenosis, spondylosis, and myeloradiculopathy by means of the posterior approach. Spine 1988;13:864–9.

[3] Mayfield FH. Cervical spondylosis: a comparison of the anterior and posterior approaches. Clin Neurosurg 1965;13:181–8.

[4] Yaeger VL, Cooper MH. Surgical anatomy of the cervical spine surrounding structures. In: Young PH, editor. Microsurgery of the cervical spine. New York: Raven Press; 1991. p. 1–17.

[5] Hirabayashi K, Watanabe S, Wakano K. Expansive open-door laminoplasty for cervical spinal stenotic myelopathy. Spine 1983;8:693–9.

[6] Hase HT, Watanabe S, Hirasawa Y. Bilateral open laminoplasty using ceramic laminas for cervical myelopathy. Spine 1991;16:1269–76.

[7] Herkowitz HN. A comparison of anterior cervical fusion, cervical laminectomy, and cervical laminoplasty for the surgical management of multiple level spondylotic radiculopathy. Spine 1988;13:774–80.

[8] Raynor RB. Anterior or posterior approach to the cervical spine: an anatomical and radiographic evaluation and comparison. Neurosurgery 1983;12(1):7–13.

[9] McAfee PC, Bohlman HH, Riley Jr LH, et al. The anterior retropharyngeal approach to the upper cervical spine. J Bone Joint Surg Am 1987;69:1371–83.

[10] Southwick WO, Robinson RA. Surgical approaches to the vertebral bodies in the cervical and lumbar regions. J Bone Joint Surg Am 1957;39:631–44.

[11] Bulger RF, Rejowski JE, Beatty RA. Vocal cord paralysis associated with anterior cervical fusion: consideration for prevention and treatment. J Neurosurg 1985;62:657–61.

[12] Regan JJ, Yuan H, McAfee PC. Laparoscopic fusion of the lumbar spine: minimally invasive spine surgery. A prospective multicenter study evaluating open and laparoscopic lumbar fusion. Spine 1999;24:402–11.

[13] Bradford DS, Zdelblick TA. Master techniques in orthopaedic surgery. In: Bradford DS, editor. The spine. New York: Lippincott Williams & Wilkins; 2004. p. 321–34.

[14] Zdeblick TA, David SM. A prospective comparison of surgical approach for anterior L4–L5 fusion: laparoscopic versus mini anterior lumbar interbody fusion. Spine 2000;25:2682–7.

[15] Bertagnoli R, Vazquez RJ. The AnteroLateral trans-Psoatic Approach (ALPA): a new technique for implanting prosthetic disk-nucleus devices. J Spinal Disord Tech 2003;16(4):398–404.

[16] Vazquez RM, Gireesan GT. Balloon-assisted endoscopic retroperitoneal gasless (BERG) technique for anterior lumbar interbody fusion (ALIF). Surg Endosc 2003;17(2):268–72.

[17] Wiltse LL. Surgery for the intervertebral disc disease of the lumbar spine. Clin Orthop 1977;129:22–45.

[18] Vialle R, Court C, Khouri N, et al. Anatomical study of the paraspinal approach to the lumbar spine. Eur Spine J 2004 [in press].

[19] Khoo LT, Palmer S, Laich DT, et al. Minimally invasive percutaneous posterior lumbar interbody fusion. Neurosurgery 2002;51(Suppl 5):166–71.

[20] Foley K, Smith M. Microendoscopic discectomy. Tech Neurosurg 1997;3:301–7.

[21] Steffee AD. The variable screw placement system with posterior lumbar interbody fusion. In: Lin PM, Gill K, editors. Lumbar interbody fusion. Rockville (MD): Aspen; 1989. p. 81–93.

[22] Steffee AD, Sitkowski DJ. Posterior lumbar interbody fusion and plates. Clin Orthop 1988;227:99–102.

[23] Branch Jr CL. Posterior lumbar interbody fusion. In: Hardy Jr RW, editor. Lumbar disc disease. 2nd edition. New York: Raven Press; 1993. p. 187–200.

[24] Brodke DS, Dick JC, Kunz DN, et al. Posterior lumbar interbody fusion: a biomechanical comparison, including a new threaded cage. Spine 1997;22:26–31.

[25] Lin PM, Cautilli RA, Joyce MF. Posterior lumbar interbody fusion. Clin Orthop 1983;180:154–68.

Lumbar Total Disc Replacement Part I: Rationale, Biomechanics, and Implant Types

Peter Frelinghuysen, MD[a,*], Russel C. Huang, MD[a,b], Federico P. Girardi, MD[a,b], Frank P. Cammisa, Jr, MD[a,b]

[a]*Hospital for Special Surgery, 535 East 70th Street, New York, NY 10021, USA*
[b]*Weill Cornell Medical College, 525 E 68th Street, New York, NY 10021, USA*

Degenerative disc disease produces back pain that is often treated by nonsurgical methods. When these methods fail, surgical treatment is offered, usually in the form of interbody fusion. The concept of eliminating the painful motion segment by discectomy and fusion is considered the "gold standard" of surgical treatment of recalcitrant degenerative disc disease; however, the results of this surgical intervention are sometimes suboptimal in terms of pain relief and associated problems such as pseudoarthrosis, iliac crest bone graft donor site pain, and adjacent-level degeneration. Total disc replacement (TDR) has been developed to preserve motion, avoid the morbidity of bone graft harvest, and possibly reduce adjacent-level degeneration. Although preliminary reports on disc replacement have been promising, it should be emphasized that until longer-term follow-up data are available, the technology should not be widely applied in lieu of fusion.

Anatomy and physiology of intervertebral disc

The intervertebral disc develops from notochordal remnants and perichordal mesenchyme. Notochordal cells may persist up to the age of 5 years and have been found in the sacral discs of older patients aged 22 to 45 years [1]. Toward the end of the embryonic period, the developing disc has an external fibrous zone, an intermediate fibrocartilaginous zone, and an internal hyaline zone adjacent to the notochord. The peripheral layers of the anulus are embedded in the outer ring of the cartilage plate, and the most external lamellae are attached to the long ligaments [2,3]. In adults, the inner gelatinous nucleus pulposus is surrounded by the fibrous outer anulus. The anulus is comprised of approximately twelve lamellae, each of which is characterized by a parallel arrangement of fibers aligned at 65° to the long axis of the spine in alternating and opposite directions. The type I collagen that makes up most of the anulus is maintained by cells that resemble fibroblasts. The nucleus, in contrast, is composed primarily of proteoglycans and type II collagen, which maintain disc turgor by their hydrophilic nature. The proteoglycan matrix is supported by cells that derive from notochord and resemble chondrocytes.

The vascularity of the disc changes with aging. At birth, the disc receives vessels that penetrate the anulus and cartilaginous end plates to supply the central nucleus pulposus. At maturity, due to gradual involution of these vessels, only the peripheral anulus receives a direct blood supply [4]. Hence, in an adult, the metabolic needs of the nucleus are met by way of diffusion. By the end of the first decade, the circumferential portion of the cartilage plate becomes

* Corresponding author.
E-mail address: frelinghuysenp@hss.edu (P. Frelinghuysen).

ossified to form the ring apophysis, with the outer annular fibers incorporated into this structure.

The innervation of the disc is much like its blood supply: the nucleus and the inner anulus are aneural. Branches of the sinuvertebral nerve, however, innervate the posterior anulus and the posterior longitudinal ligament, and density of this innervation increases with degenerative disc disease [5]. Inflammation of the disc has been shown to promote axonal regeneration of the dorsal root ganglion neurons that innervate the rat intervertebral disc [6,7]. The sinuvertebral nerve has been show to ascend or descend a level or two, and this imprecise distribution of nociceptive feedback likely contributes to the difficulty with precise localization of pain in patients who suffer degenerative disc disease. In addition, the vertebral end plates are innervated, and their degeneration may contribute to the etiology of back pain in degenerative disc disease [8,9].

Biomechanics

Given our upright posture and the load our spines must bear as a result, the human disc has evolved to handle compressive loads. The nucleus is designed to absorb compressive loads, redistribute the forces radially, and convert these forces into tensile loads in the anulus fibrosis. When disc hydration is decreased and the nucleus has suboptimal turgor, the motion segment bears the compressive load poorly, leading to shearing forces in the anulus that result in fissures and tears and the initiation of the degenerative cascade. Under normal conditions, the disc performs its tasks very well: it withstands decades of compressive, shear, and loading forces at loads up to 2.5 times body weight when walking and up to nearly 10 times body weight when lifting objects [10–12]. The anterior column of the spine bears approximately 80% of the compressive loads under normal conditions, but as the disc degenerates, an increasing amount of this responsibility is borne by the posterior structures, namely, the facets [13,14]. The posterior elements play an important role in spinal kinematics and bear careful scrutiny when considering TDR surgery. They bear high compressive loads in extension and are likely pain generators in a spondylotic spine [15,16]. The kinematics of the spinal motion segment have been well characterized and exhibit a wide variability between individuals and between different levels of the same individual [17–19]. A TDR prosthesis is unlikely to provide the exact characteristics of native anatomy; therefore, different designs can be expected to yield different long-term outcomes.

Pathophysiology of degenerative disc disease

Degenerative disc disease is nearly universal in old age and is a common phenomenon in younger patients [20,21]. As alluded to earlier, the decreased ability of the aging disc to absorb the loads associated with activities of daily living degrades the anulus and puts excess stress on the facets and end plates [22–24]. In addition to the classic, mechanical view of disc degeneration, the cellular and molecular aspects of the degenerative process and their potential genetic underpinning are being elucidated. For example, mechanical factors have been shown to directly affect the metabolic activity of disc cells. Bruehlmann et al [25] used confocal microscopy to demonstrate that collagen fibril sliding governs cell mechanics in the bovine anulus fibrosis, providing direct evidence of how mechanical loads are transferred through the extracellular matrix. Currently, it appears that the balance between the anabolic and catabolic forces in the disc is disrupted and that the degenerative process involves declining cell nutrition and viability, cell senescence, accumulation of degraded matrix molecules, overactivity of matrix metalloproteinases and aggrecanase, and hypoactivity of the tissue inhibitors of matrix proteases [26–28].

The environmental risk factors for degenerative disc disease include heavy physical work associated with lifting and awkward positions. In addition, static work postures and whole-body vibration are associated with degenerative disc disease [29,30]. In a feline model, the number of repetitions of static load on the lumbar spine was demonstrated to be a risk factor in developing lumbar cumulative trauma disorder [31].

Nonsurgical treatment

For most patients with back pain and degenerative lumbar disc disease, the treatment is nonsurgical. Most patients improve satisfactorily without surgery [32]. Modalities such as physical therapy, massage, and manipulation, have been shown to be effective [33]. In the small percentage of patients who do not benefit from nonsurgical treatment and remain disabled from their back pain, surgery can be beneficial. In a randomized trial comparing fusion with nonsurgical treatment in patients with chronic low back pain, surgery significantly improved pain levels and degree of disability [34].

Surgical treatment

The rationale for fusion as a treatment for degenerative disc disease rests on the premise that the pain generated from the painful motion segment is ameliorated by eliminating motion and loading on pathologic disc tissues. Although some surgeons have argued that a posterolateral fusion suffices, most believe that a 360° fusion, which eliminates the disc and provides solid anterior support, represents the "gold standard."

Surgical outcomes are not uniformly good, however, and the role of surgery for back pain and degenerative disc disease remains controversial. The validity of the diagnostic methodology used to determine the anatomic etiology of low back pain remains questionable [35]. In addition, a large meta-analysis showed that approximately one third of patients who had fusion surgery for low back pain and degenerative disc disease had an unsatisfactory outcome [36]. The most common complications of surgery were pseudoarthrosis, with an incidence of 16%. The second most common complication was iliac crest bone graft site pain, with an incidence of 9%. Other problems included adjacent-level disease [36]. In addition, patients often dislike and have poor compliance with postoperative bracing protocols. A recent meta-analysis showed the average fusion rate to be 85% and the average clinical success in terms of pain reduction to be 75%. It was also found that successful spinal fusion takes a relatively long time (on average, 15 months) for healing and recuperation [37].

Total disc replacement

Ideal characteristics

The ideal lumbar TDR would function as a physiologic replacement for the human intervertebral disc. It would assume the role of the nucleus pulposus and anulus fibrosis complex. In preserving the lumbar spine's range of motion, the lumbar TDR would also need to transmit and absorb loads across the disc space between the vertebral bodies. In other words, it should attempt to reproduce the load transmission properties of the disc and its motion characteristics. In addition to providing preservation of motion, the goals of disc arthroplasty include restoring disc height, foraminal height, and spinal alignment. In the perioperative period, morbidity would be reduced by avoiding bone graft site complications and postoperative bracing issues. In longer-term follow-up, an ideal TDR would eliminate the risk of pseudarthrosis and possibly reduce adjacent-level degeneration and facet degeneration. It should be noted that no class I data have confirmed that motion preservation reduces the incidence of adjacent-level disease; this "benefit" of TDR is strictly theoretic at this time. Additional benefits include shorter hospital stays and earlier return to function [38]. Given that the patient population most likely to benefit from TDR is young, the implant needs to be constructed from biocompatible materials that would prove durable for several decades in vivo.

History of total disc replacement

Although a hot topic in the modern world of spine surgery, the concept of disc replacement is not new, and the first surgical foray into the field began 40 years ago. In the 1950s, Nachemson tried implanting a silicon testicular prosthesis into the disc space but abandoned this methodology when the implants disintegrated [39]. Fernstrom [40] reported his experience of implanting a steel ball in the disc space in 1966. He began implanting ball bearings into disc spaces in the late 1950s and ultimately admitted poor results in roughly 250 patients. The balls created a segmental hypermobility and subsided through the vertebral end plates into the vertebral bodies [39]. As a result, the implant was withdrawn. There have been many attempts to create a successful intervertebral implant; the number and wide range of designs attest to the difficulty of building a device that fits into the three-joint complex of each spinal unit. In addition, unlike the hip or the knee, the disc has a damping viscoelastic component and its center of rotation changes with motion. A review of failed designs include silicon spacers alone, plastic spacers, silicon or plastic with metal end plates, various end plate designs including screws, pins, keels, cones, and even suction cups. Various diaphragms and hygroscopic agents were used in lieu of the disc, followed by elastic beads, springs, oils, and expandable gels. The few designs that have made it to the market have therefore already withstood some test of time. Szpalski et al [39] provides an excellent review of the history of spine arthroplasty surgery.

Indication and contraindications for lumbar disc arthroplasty

The indication for lumbar disc arthroplasty is back pain from degenerative disc disease in patients who have failed a protracted course of nonsurgical treatment. There are many contraindications to the use of this new technology. Spine-specific contraindications include spondylolisthesis, spondylolysis, posterior element disease (facet joint arthritis or previous facet joint resection), central or lateral recess stenosis, fixed deformity, infection, osteoporosis, or herniated nucleus pulposus with radiculopathy that cannot be decompressed by way of anterior approach. Relative contraindications include psychosocial pathology, multilevel disease, and obesity. Many of these contraindications are common in patients with degenerative disc disease. As clinical experience with TDR grows, some of these indications may be eliminated. In a review of 100 consecutive patients undergoing lumbar spine surgery for degenerative spinal disease, the prevalence of at least one contraindication to TDR was 95%. In the 56 patients in this series who underwent fusion, 100% had at least one contraindication to TDR; therefore, it is not likely that TDR will soon replace fusion in spine surgery [41].

Overview of implants types and characteristics

There are currently four lumbar total disc prostheses coming to market in the United States. The SB Charité disc (DePuy Spine/Johnson & Johnson, Raynham, Massachusetts) was approved by the Food and Drug Administration (FDA) in the fall of 2004. The ProDisc (Spine Solutions/Synthes, West Chester, Pennsylvania) has completed its randomized enrollment, is currently in nonrandomized modes, and may be approved by late 2005. The Maverick (Medtronic Sofamor Danek, Memphis, Tennessee) and FlexiCore (SpineCore/Stryker, Kalamazoo, Michigan) lumbar disc prostheses are currently actively enrolling patients with single-level disease.

ProDisc

The ProDisc was designed in the late 1980s by Thierry Marnay, a French orthopedic spine surgeon. The current design has been implanted in over 5000 patients in Europe since the late 1990s. Its design is based on spheric articulations and is composed of three components. Its metal end plates are made of cobalt-chromium-molybdenum alloy. Its central convex weight-bearing surface, which is snap fitted into the inferior end plate, is made from ultra-high molecular weight polyethylene (UHMWPE). This produces a semiconstrained device with two articulating surfaces and a fixed center of rotation. The end plates gain purchase into the vertebral bodies by means of a central keel and two spikes. The modularity of the prosthesis allows customization to match the patient's anatomy: there are two end plate sizes, three heights of polyethylene, and two different angles of lordosis.

A multicenter FDA study that began in October 2001, which included 19 centers, compared the ProDisc with 360° fusion using femoral ring allograft anteriorly with pedicle screw, rod fixation, and autograft posteriorly. The randomization protocol assigned two thirds of the patients to the ProDisc and the other third to fusion. The ProDisc was implanted at L3-4, L4-5, or L5-S1. This trial completed enrollment in April 2003 and is now awaiting completion and evaluation of the 2-year follow-up. There is also a two-level arm to the study that allows treatment at two contiguous levels from L3 through S1, and this arm of the trial completed its enrollment in November 2003 and is similarly waiting for follow-up. The ProDisc is the only prosthesis that is being evaluated by the FDA for multiple levels.

SB Charité

The SB Charité disc was approved by the FDA in November 2004. It was designed in former East Germany in the early 1980s by Shellnac and Buttner-Jans and quickly underwent two revisions to become, in 1987, the implant available today. It has two metal alloy plates and a unique separate sliding core made of UHMWPE. Theoretically, the polyethylene core can shift dynamically with spinal movement and more nearly approximate physiologic motion. The core moves posteriorly with flexion and anteriorly with extension, possibly allowing for increased motion and decreased load on the posterior facets, although this has not been clinically proved. The end plates, made of cobalt-chromium-molybdenum alloy, are affixed to the vertebral end plates by way of three anterior and two posterior teeth measuring 2.5 mm in height and are slightly recessed from the edge of the plate. The end plates are also made with a slight convexity to fit the concavity of the vertebral end plate. The biconvex UHMWPE sliding core contains a radiopaque wire. This produces an unconstrained prosthesis with a mobile center of rotation. Like the ProDisc, the Charité is modular. It comes with different sized end plates, each with different angles of lordosis and different sizes and heights of mobile cores.

The multicenter study that ultimately gained the Charité FDA approval compared the Charité with 360° fusion. In contradistinction to the ProDisc study, a threaded fusion cage was placed in the disc space anteriorly rather than allograft and no posterior surgery was performed. Again, the study protocol called for a 2:1 randomization favoring the prosthesis. The trial began in March 2000 and was approved for single-level disease at L4-5 or L5-S1. Two hundred sixty-seven discs were implanted, and the study was closed in December 2001. After 24-month follow-up and review of the data by the FDA, the Charité was approved in November 2004 by the FDA Orthopaedic and Rehabilitation Devices Panel.

Maverick

The Maverick device was conceived by Mathews et al [42] and employs a metal-on-metal ball-and-socket configuration without a polyethylene component. The cobalt-chromium end plates interface directly and use central keels to attach to the vertebral bodies. This produces a semiconstrained device with a fixed and slightly more posterior center of rotation.

The multicenter clinical trail began in the spring of 2003 and is being compared with anterior fusion using freestanding, tapered, threaded titanium lumbar tapered cages (Medtronic Sofamor Danek, Memphis, Tennessee) with Infuse (BMP-2)-soaked sponges.

Flexicore

The Flexicore device is another metal-on-metal device in which the superior and inferior portions are linked by a captured ball-and-socket joint. The device is inserted as a single unit. The end plates are domed to fit into the concavities of the vertebral bodies, are coated with a titanium plasma spray to assist in bone ingrowth fixation, and have fins that affix to the vertebral bodies. This produces a fully constrained device with a fixed center of rotation.

The multicenter trial is underway, patients with single-level disc disease are being enrolled, and the disc is being compared with 360° fusion with femoral ring allograft and posterolateral pedicle screw instrumentation and fusion with iliac crest autograft.

Surgical considerations

As is the case with any surgical procedure, it is important to have a clearly defined preoperative plan. For example, the Charité can be templated using plain radiographs and overlays of the implants much like in total joint arthroplasty. For the approach, it is critical to have an access surgeon, usually a general or vascular surgeon. In addition to the instruments required for the minimally invasive approach, it is important to have instruments available for an emergency (eg, in the event of a great vessel injury).

In general, the patient is positioned supine on a radiolucent table, and assurances of adequate C-arm fluoroscopy are confirmed. The "Da Vinci" position, with legs and arms spread, allows the surgeon to operate from between the legs. Pulse oximetry of the left great toe can help prevent overzealous retraction of the left iliac artery. With stretching and manipulation of the left common and external iliac artery, decreased oxygen saturation by oximetry may be the first sign of vascular injury.

The surgical approach varies depending on the level. A Pfannenstiel skin incision for the L5-S1 segment is suitable, but for the upper lumbar levels, a longitudinal (midline or paramedian) incision is necessary. The retroperitoneal approach is preferred. After incising the skin and the subcutaneous tissue, the surgeon should expose the linea alba and continue, bluntly exposing laterally to the left to expose the anterior rectus sheath, which is then incised longitudinally and retracted laterally. Blunt dissection is used again to develop the plane between the posterior aspect of the posterior rectus sheath and the peritoneum, followed by a longitudinal incision of the posterior rectus sheath as necessary. The retroperitoneal fat tissue is assuaged with sponge sticks and, using the psoas as a lateral guide, dissection proceeds rightward to the lumbar spine. The ureter, if encountered, is retracted to the right with the peritoneum. When approaching the L5-S1 disc space, working distal to the bifurcation of the great vessels, it is important to expose and control the median sacral artery and vein that cross the disc space. When approaching the L4-L5 disc space, one encounters the lateral aspect of the disc at the medial margin of the left psoas. The sympathetic trunk is identified and dissected free. The major vessels are then mobilized rightward, taking care to identify and, if needed, ligate the ascending lumbar vein that drains into the left common iliac vein. For L3-L4 and above, the vascular dissection is less arduous, usually only requiring ligation of the segmental vessels. After the disc space is exposed, radiography is used to confirm the level. Retractors are placed to assure adequate working space and to protect critical neighboring structures. The anulus is incised, and the disc is removed using rongeurs, leaving the lateral anulus intact. The cartilaginous end plates are carefully removed, making sure to preserve the integrity of the bony end plates to help prevent subsidence. Osteophytes that might prevent proper implant positioning are removed. For some implants, like the Charité, distraction of the vertebral bodies is required to clear the teeth. For other implants, like the ProDisc, preparation of the bodies for the keel is required using a specially designed osteotome. In all cases, attention to alignment is critical. A sizing device is used to determine the appropriate component size; it is important to keep the implants on the smaller size (ie, avoid overstuffing the disc space). In contrast to anterior lumbar interbody fusion whereby large implants are used to create tension in ligamentous and annular structures for the purpose of enhancing stability, in arthroplasty, smaller implants may help preserve motion.

Postoperative regime

Similar to the patient education programs used for joint arthroplasty, the authors believe that preoperative education is beneficial. Studies have shown that early mobilization is better [43]. Early motion is best limited to flexion, and no rotation should be allowed for at least 3 weeks. At 6 weeks, the patient can be advanced to rotation and side bending. After 6 weeks, the patient can extend past neutral and begin abdominal exercises. Some advocate a soft brace until that time, recommending avoidance of extremes of motion until out of the brace. If all goes well, a return to sports is allowable at 3 months.

Summary

The excitement surrounding TDR surgery must be tempered with prudence. Motion preservation surgery of the spine is still in its early stages, and although the clinical results are promising, the complexity of the functional spinal unit exceeds the designs of the current implants. Exacting indications, careful surgical technique, and thorough follow-up will allow us to improve on this promising beginning.

References

[1] Wolfe HJ, Putschar WG, Vickery AL. Role of the notochord in human intervetebral disk. I. Fetus and infant. Clin Orthop 1965;39:205–12.

[2] Walmsley R. The development and growth of the intervertebral disc. Edinburgh Med J 1953;60:341–64.

[3] Hickey DS, Hukins DW. X-ray diffraction studies of the arrangement of collagenous fibres in human fetal intervertebral disc. J Anat 1980;131:81–90.

[4] Whalen JL, Parke WW, Mazur JM, et al. The intrinsic vasculature of developing vertebral end plates and its nutritive significance to the intervertebral discs. J Pediatr Orthop 1985;5:403–10.

[5] Coppes MH, Marani E, Thomeer RT, et al. Innervation of "painful" lumbar discs. Spine 1997;22:2342–50.

[6] Aoki Y, Ohtori S, Ino H, et al. Disc inflammation potentially promotes axonal regeneration of dorsal root ganglion neurons innervating lumbar intervertebral disc in rats. Spine 2004;29:2621–6.

[7] Aoki Y, Ohtori S, Takahashi K, et al. Innervation of the lumbar intervertebral disc by nerve growth factor-dependent neurons related to inflammatory pain. Spine 2004;29:1077–81.

[8] Antonacci MD, Mody DR, Heggeness MH. Innervation of the human vertebral body: a histologic study. J Spinal Disord 1998;11:526–31.

[9] Brown MF, Hukkanen MV, McCarthy ID, et al. Sensory and sympathetic innervation of the vertebral endplate in patients with degenerative disc disease. J Bone Joint Surg Br 1997;79:147–53.

[10] Cappozzo A. Compressive loads in the lumbar vertebral column during normal level walking. J Orthop Res 1984;1:292–301.

[11] Granata KP, Marras WS, Davis KG. Variation in spinal load and trunk dynamics during repeated lifting exertions. Clin Biomech (Bristol, Avon) 1999;14:367–75.

[12] Sparto PJ, Parnianpour M. Estimation of trunk muscle forces and spinal loads during fatiguing repetitive trunk exertions. Spine 1998;23:2563–73.

[13] Bergmark A. Stability of the lumbar spine. A study in mechanical engineering. Acta Orthop Scand Suppl 1989;230:1–54.

[14] Cunningham BW, Kotani Y, McNulty PS, et al. The effect of spinal destabilization and instrumentation on lumbar intradiscal pressure: an in vitro biomechanical analysis. Spine 1997;22:2655–63.

[15] Cavanaugh JM, Ozaktay AC, Yamashita HT, et al. Lumbar facet pain: biomechanics, neuroanatomy and neurophysiology. J Biomech 1996;29:1117–29.

[16] Dreyer SJ, Dreyfuss PH. Low back pain and the zygapophysial (facet) joints. Arch Phys Med Rehabil 1996;77:290–300.

[17] Gertzbein SD, Holtby R, Tile M, et al. Determination of a locus of instantaneous centers of rotation of the lumbar disc by moire fringes. A new technique. Spine 1984;9:409–13.

[18] Pearcy MJ, Bogduk N. Instantaneous axes of rotation of the lumbar intervertebral joints. Spine 1988;13:1033–41.

[19] Yoshioka T, Tsuji H, Hirano N, et al. Motion characteristic of the normal lumbar spine in young adults: instantaneous axis of rotation and vertebral center motion analyses. J Spinal Disord 1990;3:103–13.

[20] Boden SD, Davis DO, Dina TS, et al. Abnormal magnetic-resonance scans of the lumbar spine in asymptomatic subjects. A prospective investigation. J Bone Joint Surg Am 1990;72:403–8.

[21] Boden SD, McCowin PR, Davis DO, et al. Abnormal magnetic-resonance scans of the cervical spine in asymptomatic subjects. A prospective investigation. J Bone Joint Surg Am 1990;72:1178–84.

[22] Modic MT, Masaryk TJ, Ross JS, et al. Imaging of degenerative disk disease. Radiology 1988;168:177–86.

[23] Modic MT, Steinberg PM, Ross JS, et al. Degenerative disk disease: assessment of changes in vertebral body marrow with MR imaging. Radiology 1988;166:193–9.

[24] Panjabi MM, Krag MH, Chung TQ. Effects of disc injury on mechanical behavior of the human spine. Spine 1984;9:707–13.

[25] Bruehlmann SB, Matyas JR, Duncan NA. ISSLS Prize Winner: collagen fibril sliding governs cell mechanics in the anulus fibrosus: an in situ confocal microscopy study of bovine discs. Spine 2004;29:2612–20.

[26] Buckwalter JA. Aging and degeneration of the human intervertebral disc. Spine 1995;20:1307–14.

[27] Gruber HE, Hanley Jr EN. Analysis of aging and degeneration of the human intervertebral disc. Comparison of surgical specimens with normal controls. Spine 1998;23:751–7.

[28] Roberts S, Caterson B, Menage J, et al. Matrix metalloproteinases and aggrecanase: their role in disorders of the human intervertebral disc. Spine 2000;25:3005–13.

[29] Pope MH. Degenerative disc disease and occupational exposure. 1st edition. Philadelphia: Lippincot Williams & Wilkins; 2004. p. 35–52.

[30] Pope MH, Goh KL, Magnusson ML. Spine ergonomics. Annu Rev Biomed Eng 2002;4:49–68.

[31] Sbriccoli P, Yousuf K, Kupershtein I, et al. Static load repetition is a risk factor in the development of lumbar cumulative musculoskeletal disorder. Spine 2004;29:2643–53.

[32] Atlas SJ, Nardin RA. Evaluation and treatment of low back pain: an evidence-based approach to clinical care. Muscle Nerve 2003;27:265–84.

[33] Cherkin DC, Sherman KJ, Deyo RA, et al. A review of the evidence for the effectiveness, safety, and cost of acupuncture, massage therapy, and spinal manipulation for back pain. Ann Intern Med 2003;138:898–906.

[34] Fritzell P, Hagg O, Wessberg P, et al. 2001 Volvo Award Winner in Clinical Studies: lumbar fusion versus nonsurgical treatment for chronic low back pain: a multicenter randomized controlled trial from the Swedish Lumbar Spine Study Group. Spine 2001;26:2521–34.

[35] Saal JS. General principles of diagnostic testing as related to painful lumbar spine disorders: a critical appraisal of current diagnostic techniques. Spine 2002;27:2538–46.

[36] Turner JA, Ersek M, Herron L, et al. Patient outcomes after lumbar spinal fusions. JAMA 1992;268:907–11.

[37] Bono CM, Lee CK. Critical analysis of trends in fusion for degenerative disc disease over the past 20 years: influence of technique on fusion rate and clinical outcome. Spine 2004;29:455–63.

[38] Anderson PA, Rouleau JP. Intervertebral disc arthroplasty. Spine 2004;29:2779–86.

[39] Szpalski M, Gunzburg R, Mayer M. Spine arthroplasty: a historical review. Eur Spine J 2002;11(Suppl 2):S65–84.

[40] Fernstrom U. Arthroplasty with intercorporal endoprothesis in herniated disc and in painful disc. Acta Chir Scand Suppl 1966;357:154–9.

[41] Huang RC, Lim MR, Girardi FP, et al. The prevalence of contraindications to total disc replacement in a cohort of lumbar surgical patients. Spine 2004;29:2538.

[42] Mathews HH, Lehuec JC, Friesem T, et al. Design rationale and biomechanics of Maverick total disc arthroplasty with early clinical results. Spine J 2004;4:S268–75.

[43] Cinotti G, David T, Postacchini F. Results of disc prosthesis after a minimum follow-up period of 2 years. Spine 1996;21:995–1000.

Clinical Results of ProDisc-II Lumbar Total Disc Replacement: Report from the United States Clinical Trial

Rick B. Delamarter, MD, Hyun W. Bae, MD, Ben B. Pradhan, MD, MSE*

Spine Research Foundation, The Spine Institute at Saint John's Health Center, Suite 400, 1301 20th Street, Santa Monica, CA 90404, USA

Chronic low back pain from degenerative disc disease is endemic in our society. The surgical treatment of this problem can often be frustrating. Fusion of the painful degenerative segment is often associated with mediocre results, prolonged recovery time, significant postoperative morbidity, and future degeneration at the adjacent levels. Lumbar disc replacement has been shown to be a promising alternative in the treatment of low back pain and may eliminate the stigmas associated with fusion. The long track record of lumbar disc replacements in Europe combined with the recently completed United States Investigational Device Exemption (US IDE) pivotal clinical trials have provided encouraging results for this motion-preservation technology compared with spinal fusion. Interest in disc replacement has risen rapidly in the last few years in the United States, but the concept itself is not new. It represents the latest development in the spectrum of nonfusion surgical technologies for spinal reconstruction.

Despite the controversy surrounding surgical fusion of the painful degenerating functional spinal unit, for lack of a better alternative it has de facto become the "gold standard" procedure for intractable cases that fail nonoperative treatment. The specter of potential complications and poor outcomes from fusion has however driven a major effort to develop numerous motion-preserving anterior or posterior spinal column reconstruction techniques. Conceptually, the logical progression of intervention for a degenerative spinal segment should be as depicted in Fig. 1, with examples of currently available state-of-the-art implants at each stage. Each subsequent intervention can be considered a salvage procedure for the previous procedure. Dynamic neutralization and nucleus replacement may be performed individually or in combination. These devices are still considered experimental pending the completion of clinical trials. A spinal fusion, the present gold standard, is still available as the end-stage salvage procedure.

The ProDisc implant

Thierry Marnay created the first ProDisc-I prosthetic disc in 1989 at Montpellier, France. The first human implantation was in 1990. To his credit, after implanting 93 implants in almost 70 patients, Marnay stopped to evaluate the long-term outcomes of his implant. Finally, in 2001 and 2005 he published his results after an 8- to 10-year follow-up [1–3]. All implants remained intact without any migration or subsidence. Range of motion of the spinal segments was maintained. Back and leg pain were significantly reduced, and almost 93% of the patients were satisfied and would have the surgery again. The promising results from his experience paved the way for the pivotal clinical trials recently completed in the United States.

The first generation ProDisc-I had titanium endplates and a double keel. In 1999, it was changed to cobalt chrome endplates with a single keel (ProDisc-II, Fig. 2). The single serrated keel over each endplate, two small lateral pegs, along with the plasma-sprayed ingrowth surface give the implant

---

* Corresponding author.
E-mail address: bpradhanb@hotmail.com (B.B. Pradhan).

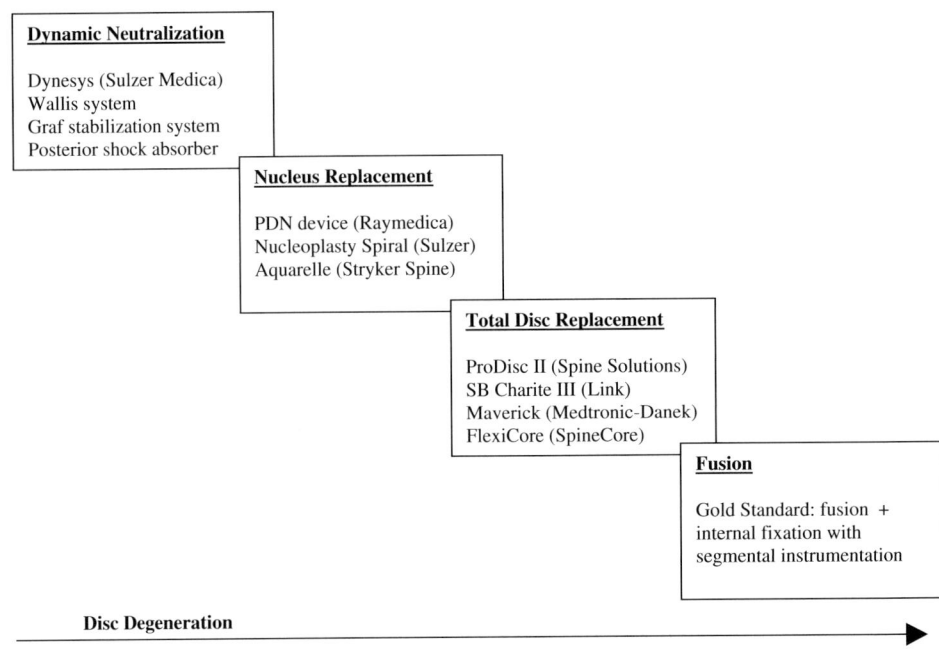

Fig. 1. Options in surgical treatment of degenerative disc disease.

immediate stability. The insert is made of ultra-high molecular weight polyethylene, which snap-locks to the bottom endplate and thus has only one articulating convex side. The device is semiconstrained, allowing it to "load-share" with collateral structures such as the facet joints, ligaments, tendons, and muscles, especially in shear. This places more load at the device-bone interface but protects the facet joints. Axial rotation is unconstrained, and the axis of rotation of the cephalad endplate is angled posteriorly in the neutral position due to the intradiscal lordosis of the prosthesis, consistent with the physiologic axis of rotation [4].

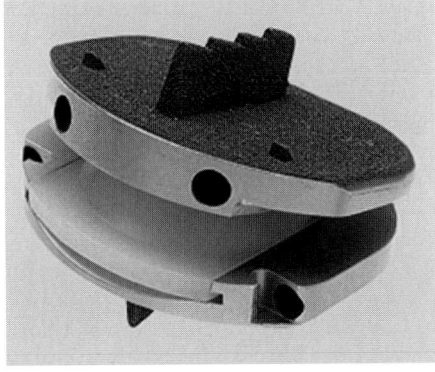

Fig. 2. The ProDisc-II (Synthes, Paoli, PA).

At the time of article submission, more than 5000 ProDisc-II prostheses have been implanted worldwide since 1999 [5]. A body of literature on the outcomes of these procedures already exists and is listed in Table 1. In general, results have been favorable, with outcomes consistently in the 90% good to excellent results, and with significant decreases in pain and disability scores. Functionally speaking, in the experience at our institute, the disc replacement patients had significantly greater segmental range of motion compared with the controlled fusion group at up to 24 months. [6,7] Bertagnoli and Kumar [8] reported an average range of motion of 10 degrees at L3-L4, L4-L5 and 9 degrees at L5-S1 at 1 year after ProDisc placement. Tropiano et al [9] reported a 10 degree range of motion at L4-L5 and 8 degree range of motion L5-S1 after a mean of 1.4 years of follow-up. Huang et al [10] reported that at a mean of 8.7 years, the ProDisc prostheses had a mean measurable motion of 4 degrees at L3-L4, 4.5 degrees at L4-L5, and 3.2 degrees at L5-S1 without any radiographic evidence of loosening or osteolysis. Equally important, only nine of 34 (26%) junctional levels above the prostheses demonstrated transitional degeneration at a mean of 8.7 years, none of them requiring surgery. In a comparable follow-up period, Cauchoix and David [11] reported transitional changes in 79% of patients 10 years after fusion surgery. For a follow-up ranging from

Table 1
ProDisc outcome studies

Study	Number of patients (N)	Mean follow-up in years	Results (% good/excellent)
Marnay [1]	64	7–11	93%
Mayer and Wiechert [19]	34	0.5	83%
Marnay [2]	>200	2	Favorable early results
Bertagnoli and Kumar [8]	108	Up to 2	99%
Delamarter et al [6]	35	0.5	Significantly lower VAS, ODS
Zigler et al [14]	49	0.4	Significantly lower VAS, ODS
Tropiano et al [9]	53	1.4	94%
Bae et al [7]	56	1.5–2	Significantly lower VAS, ODS

Abbreviations: ODS, Oswestry Disability Score; VAS, Visual Analog Score.

2 to 15 years, Gillet [12] reported transitional degeneration in 32% after 1-level fusion, but severe enough for 11% to need further surgery.

There are few published reports of device or insert subluxation, dislocation, migration, or subsidence. This is likely due to the uniconvex articular surface of the polyethylene insert, fixation of the insert to the lower endplate, and the larger serrated keels on the endplates. The insert locks onto the lower metal endplate. The surgeon needs to make sure it is snapped on flush, for an error in this step, though uncommon, can risk it coming loose. Mayer et al [13] described one patient in a series of 34 patients who underwent reoperation to replace an insert that wasn't locked into place properly. Similarly, Zigler et al [14] describe one case out of 28 where the insert was not locked in properly. Tropiano et al [9] described two cases of malposition of the implant at time of surgery in a series of 53, with three patients needing reoperation.

United States pivotal clinical trial

Currently, 19 US sites are participating in a large-scale, prospective, randomized study comparing clinical outcomes between patients receiving circumferential fusions and the ProDisc-II total disc replacement for one- and two-level degenerative disc disease in the lumbosacral spine L3-S1 vertebral segments. This study is a US Food and Drug Administration (FDA) Investigational Device Exemption multicenter, prospective, randomized study to investigate the safety and efficacy of this ProDisc-II implant. The current enrollment goal was 500 patients, which has been surpassed with surgeries falling under "continued access" or "compassionate use" arrangements with the FDA. Such arrangements have been allowed because of the promising early clinical results achieved by patients receiving the artificial discs. This is an interim comparative analysis and description of the first 78 randomized patients at 2 years after ProDisc total disc replacement or anterior/posterior fusion from one site participating in the FDA-regulated IDE study (ProDisc investigational device exemption #G010133, Synthes, NY).

Design

Approval to conduct the study was given by the FDA and by our participating center's Institutional Review Board (IRB). Patients with predominantly back pain and one or two levels of lumbar degenerative disc disease were considered for the study. Patients were evaluated with plain radiographs, MRI, and occasionally discogram/CT scans. Meticulous inclusion and exclusion criteria were applied and are listed in Table 2. After all criteria were met, the patient was randomized to either anterior-posterior fusion with femoral allograft in the front and autologous iliac crest bone graft with instrumentation in the back, or total disc replacement through an anterior retroperitoneal approach. The randomization was performed such that two out of three patients would receive the prosthetic disc and one out of three would receive circumferential fusion. The circumferential fusion was the current standard of care for up to two-level degenerative disc disease. Patients were blinded to the treatment until after the surgical procedure was performed.

Surgical technique for the ProDisc-II

The ProDisc-II is implanted via an anterior approach to the lumbar spine. In our institute, we use the anterior retroperitoneal approach with a mini-incision less than 6 cm for one-level cases and about 8 cm for two-levels. Intraoperative fluoroscopy is used throughout the operation to verify the placement of the prosthesis. Once exposure is obtained, an anteroposterior (AP) view confirms the level and identifies the midline, which is then marked with the

Table 2
Criteria for patient enrollment in the USA ProDisc-II clinical trial

Inclusion criteria	Exclusion criteria
Degenerative disc disease in one or two adjacent levels between L3-S1	More than two levels of degenerative disc disease
	Endplate dimensions less than 34.5 mm medial-lateral or 27 mm anteroposterior
Back and/or leg pain	Known metal and/or polyethylene allergies
Failure of at least 6 months of conservative therapy	Prior lumbar fusion surgery
Oswestry score >20/50 (>40%)	Clinically compromised vertebral bodies due to prior trauma
Ability to comply with protocol and follow-up	Clinically significant degenerative facet disease
Ability to give informed consent	Lytic spondylolisthesis and/or clinically significant stenosis
Radiographic evidence of disc degeneration includes	Degenerative spondylolisthesis >grade I
1. Decrease in disc height by at least 2 mm	Back or leg pain of unknown etiology
2. Instability indicated by >3 mm translation or >5 degrees of angulation, but less than grade I slip	Objective diagnosis of osteoporosis (DEXA scan)
	Presence of metabolic bone disease (eg, Paget's, osteomalacia)
3. Annular thickening and disc desiccation on MRI	Morbid obesity (Body Mass Index >40)
4. Herniated nucleus pulposus	Pregnancy or expected pregnancy within 3 years
5. Vacuum phenomenon	Active infection
	Medications that retard healing (eg, steroids)
	Autoimmune diseases (eg, rheumatoid arthritis)
	Systemic diseases (eg, AIDS, HIV, hepatitis)
	Active malignancy

cautery. A complete diskectomy is then performed. Cartilage is removed from the vertebral endplates. If herniated disc material is identified on the preoperative MRI, this may be removed through the anterior approach. In some cases, the posterior longitudinal ligament may have contracted, preventing re-expansion of the disc space, so this must be released from the posterior vertebral body with a forward-angled curette. Once the normal anatomic height has been restored with distraction under fluoroscopy, a trial is placed to help select the proper disc size, angle, and height. A sagittal groove is then cut in the vertebral endplates in the exact midline, using a chisel placed over the trial. This groove will accept the central keel of the implant. The trial is removed, and the final implant is then securely impacted into place with an insertion tool. The insertion tool allows distraction of the disc space for placement of the UHMWPE liner, which is snap-fit into position. After the insertion instrument is removed, gross inspection is made to ensure the UHMWPE liner is properly flush against the inferior endplate (Fig. 3), and final fluoroscopic views are taken to confirm correct position of the prosthesis (Fig. 4).

Surgical technique for circumferential fusion

The same anterior approach is used for the anterior diskectomy and fusion. The endplates are also prepared in the same manner, except a femoral ring allograft is placed in the intervertebral space instead of the prosthesis. A standard technique is used for the posterior pedicle screw instrumentation and fusion. The iliac crest bone graft is taken through a separate incision.

Outcome instruments

Patients were asked to complete the standardized Oswestry Disability Index questionnaires [15,16] and to rate their pain on the Visual Analog Scale (VAS) before surgery and at each follow-up clinic visit (6 weeks, 3 months, 6 months, 12 months,

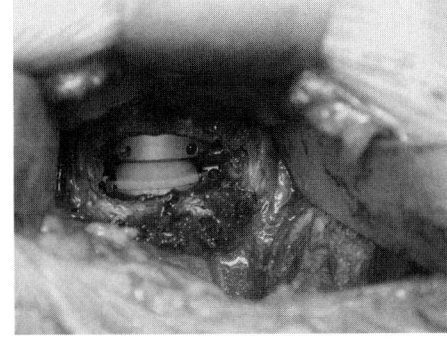

Fig. 3. The polyethylene insert must be flush and locked against the inferior plate.

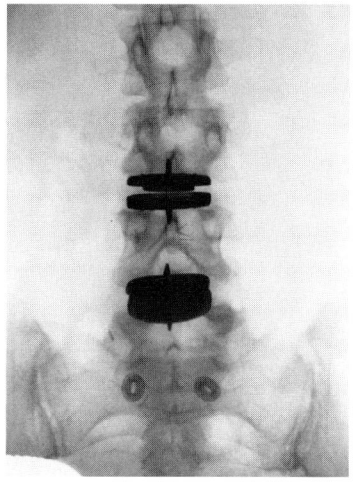 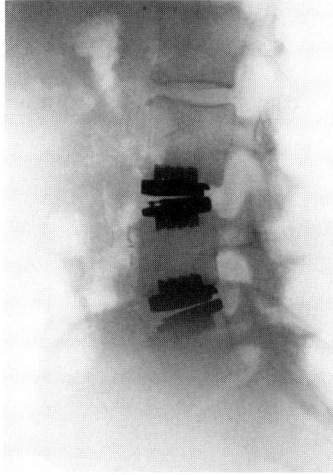

Fig. 4. Final intraoperative fluoroscopic views are inspected to confirm correct positions of prostheses.

18 months, and 24 months). On the follow-up assessments, each patient was requested to remember the pain felt before surgery and asked, "Remembering the pain you felt before surgery, would you have this surgery again?" Additionally, a 10-cm line visual scale (similar to the VAS) was presented to the patient with the instruction to "indicate the amount of satisfaction you feel with your treatment." Investigator-initiated structured queries were on types of recreational activity, ambulatory status, and medications taken for pain.

Radiographs

Flexion, extension, anteroposterior, lateral, and lateral side-to-side bending radiographs (six views total) were taken before surgery and after surgery at 6 weeks, 3, 6, 12, 18, 24 months, and annually thereafter for the artificial disc replacement patients. For fusion patients, only AP and lateral films were taken at 6 weeks and 3 months. At the 6-month and all subsequent postoperative visits, all six radiographs were taken for them as well.

Statistical analysis

Outcomes, range of motion, and demographics were analyzed statistically. Outcome measures and motion data were analyzed by using mixed designs analysis of variance (ANOVA) with repeated measures for assessment interval and a grouping effect for treatment modality (SAS, GLM procedures). Student t-tests and χ^2 were used for simple comparisons across treatments. To determine specific effects, post hoc pair-wise statistical comparisons were made with Student t-tests (group) or paired t-tests (interval within subjects). Angular range of motion was measured at L3-L4, L4-L5, and L5-S1 segments in flexion-extension, and right and left lateral bending. Analysis of variance equations were computed on degrees of motion data including a grouping effect for treatment and within effect for assessment interval,

Table 3
Characteristics of randomized patients treated with artificial discs versus those treated with fusion

Subject characteristics	Treatment		P value
	Disc replacement (n = 56)	Fusion (n = 22)	
Gender (% male)	57%	45%	not significant
Age (average years and range)	39.7 (19–59)	44.2 (25–59)	not significant
Smoking currently	11%	23%	not significant
Worker's compensation cases	33%	39%	not significant
One-level surgery	21	5	
Two-level surgery	35	17	

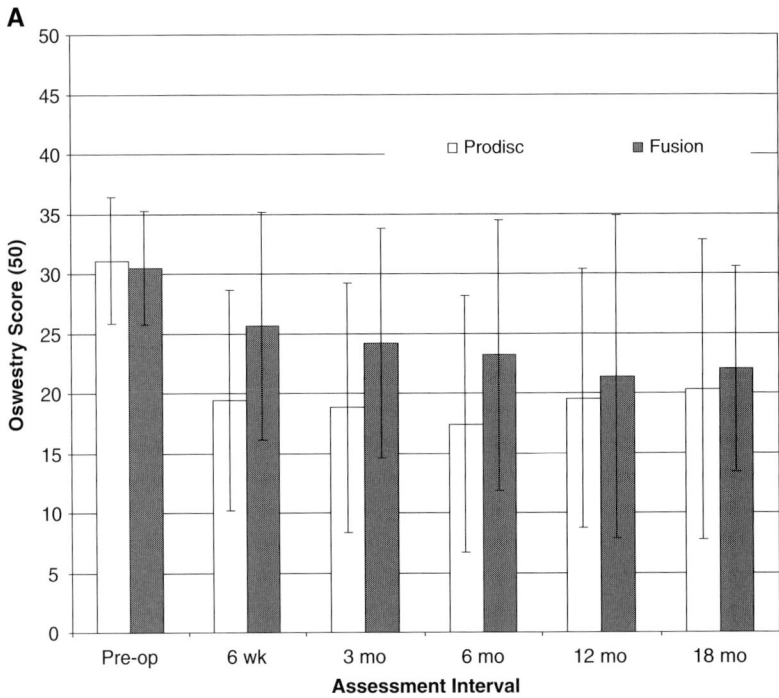
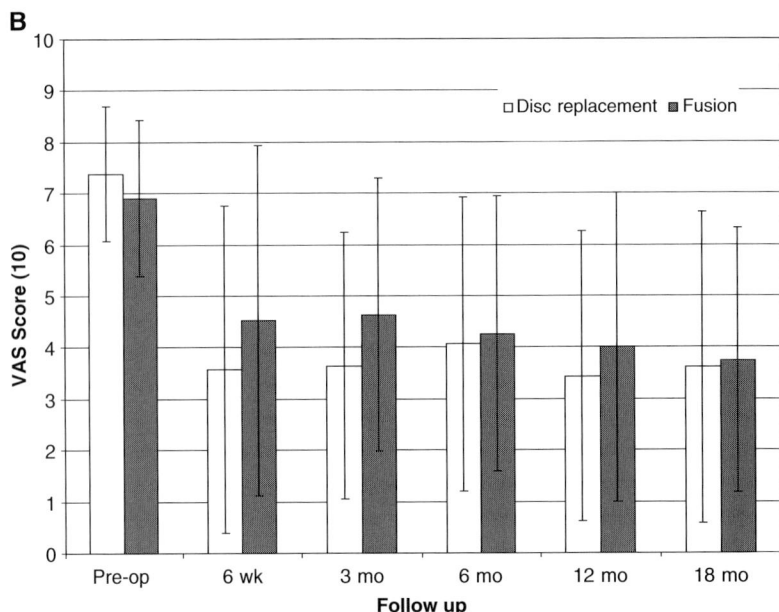

Fig. 5. (*A*) Mean and standard deviations of disability as measured by the Oswestry Questionnaire for patients treated with artificial disc compared with those treated with a fusion procedure. (*B*) Mean and standard deviations of pain as measured by the Visual Analog Scale (10-cm line) for patients treated with artificial disc compared with those treated with a fusion procedure. (*C*) A significantly higher percentage of patients were satisfied with their artificial disc replacement surgeries compared with fusion patients.

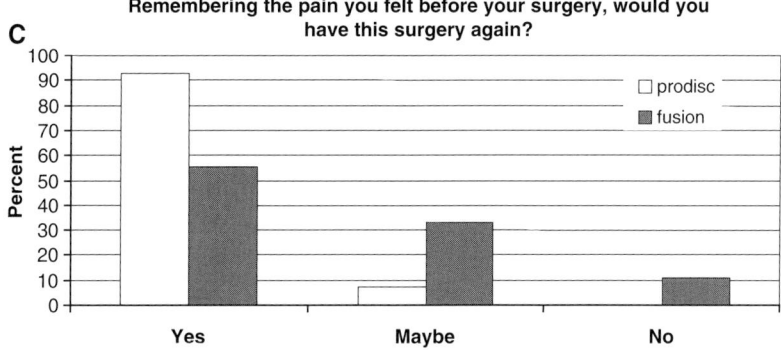

Fig. 5 (*continued*).

separately for each treated segment (L3-L4, L4-L5, and L5-S1).

Results

Data from the first 78 randomized patients (56 ProDisc-II and 22 fusion) with 18- to 24-month follow-up were available for interim analysis. The average age, gender, narcotic use, smoking history, worker's compensation percentage, and duration of back pain before surgery was similar between patients treated with artificial disc replacement (DR) and those treated with a spinal fusion (F), presented in Table 3. Of the 26 patients that were treated for one-level disc disease, there were 21 patients who had disc replacement procedures and five patients who had fusion procedures. Of the 52 patients treated who had two-level disease, 35 patients had disc replacement and 17 patients had fusion procedures. There were no instances of implant migration, breakage, or mechanical failure, nor was any revision surgery required.

Outcome measures

Preoperative values on the VAS and Oswestry Disability Index (ODI) were not significantly different among patients randomized to disc replacement or fusion. After treatment, the disc replacement patients had significantly better results at 6 weeks (VAS) and 3 months (VAS, ODI) compared with fusion patients. By 6 months, although both treatment groups showed significant improvement compared with preoperative values, there was no longer a significant difference between the two groups. From 6 months out to 2 years, the disc replacement patients continued to show more improvement than fusion patients, but the difference was not significant. At the longest follow-up, both groups were significantly improved from their preoperative state (Fig. 5A–C).

Patients who received a disc replacement had a significant decrease in pain as measured by the VAS as early as 6 weeks after surgery ($P<0.05$). At 3-month, 6-month, 12-month, 18-month, and 24-month intervals, this significant reduction in pain was maintained at about a 50% decrease from preoperative levels (all P values <0.05). Fusion patients also showed significant improvement in VAS scores postoperatively versus preoperatively ($P<0.05$). A direct comparison between the groups of patients revealed disc replacement treated patients had significantly less pain than fusion treated patients at 3 months ($P<0.05$).

The patients treated with the disc replacement also reported quicker increase in functional ability than those who underwent spinal fusion (Table 4). Disability was significantly reduced from preoperative reports (ODI) for disc replacement patients by as early as 3 months ($P<0.001$). It took fusion patients generally 6 months before a significant improvement was observed ($P<0.01$). Disc replacement patients had significantly more reduction in early pain and disability. At 6 months and later up to 2 years,

Table 4
Average recovery rates of disc replacement patients

	Treatment	
Functional status	One-level disc replacement	Two-level disc
Hospital stay	2 days	3 days
Return to work	2 weeks	2–3 weeks
Recreational sports	3 months	3 months

disc replacement and fusion patients had similar scores on both the VAS and ODI. At final follow-up, 93% of the patients reported that they were "satisfied" or "entirely satisfied" with the procedure.

Estimated motion from flexion-extension radiographs

Range of motion data are presented separately for treated vertebral segments L4-L5 (Fig. 6A) and for L5-S1 (Fig. 6B). Flexion-extension angular differences measured from radiographs yielded a measure of estimated range of motion. Motion for the disc replacement and fusion-treated segments are presented for preoperative and postoperative intervals (6 months and 12 months). Flexion-extension radiographs were not obtained after surgery for fusion patients until the 6-month follow-up visit.

An analysis of sagittal angular motion revealed an increase in motion from preoperative to the 6-month postoperative period for the L4-L5 vertebral segment

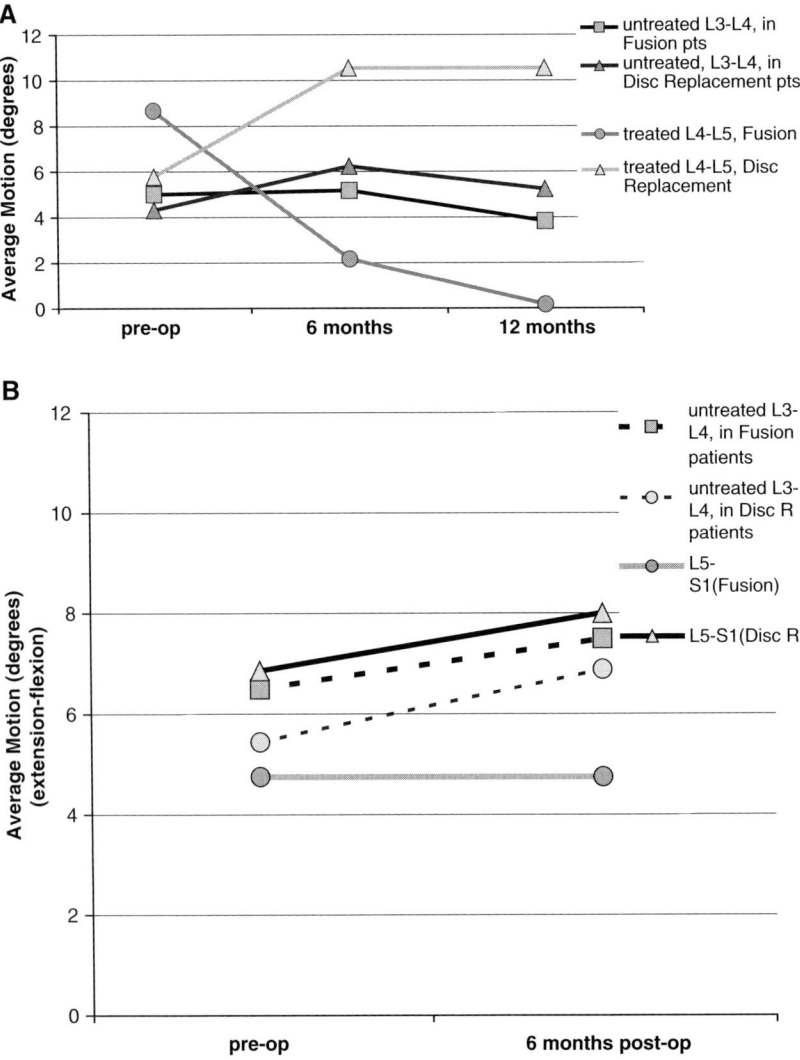

Fig. 6. (*A*) Means for motion at the L4-L5 segment and the L3-L4 segment for patients treated at the L4-L5 segment with artificial disc versus fusion. Motion was determined from flexion-extension angular measurements. (*B*) Means for motion at the L5-S1 segment and the L3-L4 segment for patients treated at the L4-L5 segment with artificial disc versus fusion. Motion was determined from flexion-extension angular measurements (1–2 year data are available but were still being measured from radiographs at time of this printing).

in patients treated at L4-L5 with the disc replacement. This motion was maintained at the 12-month period. Conversely, patients who had a fusion at L4-L5 had a significant decrease in motion from the preoperative to the 6-month period, and this trended to no motion toward 12 months out. Significantly greater motion was found at L4-L5 for disc replacement patients compared with fusion patients ($P<0.05$ at all time points). The 6-month (see Fig. 6B) and 12-month results for the L5-S1 treated segments had a similar trend, as there is increased motion at the L5-S1 level in disc replacement patients and less motion in fusion patients, although this difference is not statistically significant.

For an evaluation of consistency in the methodology used to compute motion from radiographic measurements, data from the untreated L3-L4 segments were evaluated separately in each group. There was no significant difference in angular motion at the untreated L3-L4 level measured before surgery and after surgery at 6 months and 12 months for patients in the disc replacement or fusion group. Fig. 6A presents L3-L4 data for patients treated at L4-L5, and Fig. 6B presents L3-L4 data for patients treated at L5-S1 (no significant difference).

Discussion

Demonstration of superiority or at least equivalency to the current standard of care is a prerequisite for new treatments in degenerative disc disease to be accepted in practice. Although lumbar spinal fusion has led to some improvement in symptoms compared with nonsurgical care, unfortunately many patients continue to have pain and functional limitations. Smith et al [17] showed a 68% clinical improvement at 5 years in 25 patients suffering from low back pain and who had positive discograms but refused surgical intervention. One of the most acclaimed recent studies on fusion for low back pain revealed that 60% to 68% of patients rated themselves "better" or "much better" at 2 years after surgery, and 12% to 16% were "worse" [18]. VAS scores decreased from 6 to 4 on average, and leg pain decreased from 4 to 3. Overall Fritzell et al [18] showed that lumbar fusion reduced back pain by 33% compared with 7% with nonsurgical treatment. In this study, disability according to the ODI was reduced by 25% compared with 6% in the nonsurgical patients.

In comparison with published results from lumbar spinal fusion for chronic low back pain, the initial European study on the ProDisc prosthesis showed more promise. A retrospective study of the original ProDisc-I, with 7 to 11 years of follow-up on 61 patients was conducted [1]. One third of these patients had two-level ProDisc-I implantation. There were no cases of subsidence or migration, and no implants had to be removed or revised. Overall, 92.7% of the patients reported that they were "satisfied" or "entirely satisfied" with the procedure. The average VAS for back pain went from 8.5 to 3.0 from pre-op to post-op. VAS for leg pain went from 7.0 pre-op to 2.0 post-op.

The excellent European results with the ProDisc devices with the lack of any catastrophic failures or device-related issues have paved the way for the FDA pivotal clinical trials currently underway in the United States. The interim results presented here are derived from the subset of all patients with 18 to 24 months of follow-up at a single institution. Although this analysis is limited to one site in the US trial and represents a mid-term report, it does provide prospective information on how randomized patients recover after prosthetic disc replacement versus fusion procedures in the postoperative period up to 2 years. Disc replacement patients display less pain on the VAS at the early postoperative period up to 6 months and have significantly improved functional status (lower ODI) at up to 6 months compared with fusion patients.

The early superiority of disc replacement over fusion may be partially explained by the decreased postsurgical morbidity in the disc replacement group. Disc replacement patients have only an anterior procedure and thus do not have to recover from the additional posterior approach and harvesting of iliac crest bone graft necessary for spinal fusion. Circumferential spinal fusion (as opposed to anterior only) was chosen as the "standard of care" controls because the ProDisc-II is unique among the proposed artificial disc designs in the market today in that it can be used for two-level degenerative disc disease. Standalone anterior spinal fusion is not the standard of care for multilevel degenerative disc disease.

Fusion patients did not report a significant increase in functional status and decrease in pain until the 6-month period. At the 6-month assessment, they had similar VAS and ODI scores to the disc replacement patients, showing a marked improvement from 3 to 6 months. Compared with their pre-op status, the spinal fusion patients also had dramatic improvement in their VAS and ODI scores by 6 months. This may be due to consolidation of the fusion. However, this may also be partially explained by a selection bias, because all patients in this study have to meet strict selection criteria before qualifying for the study (Table 2).

The issue of motion preservation was critically evaluated from pre-op to 24 months in both disc replacement and fusion patients. All patients in this motion analysis were treated at either the L4-L5 or L5-S1 level, or both. At the L5-S1 level, an increase in sagittal motion in the disc replacement patients was observed compared with fusion patients. However, this difference was not significantly different. This may be in part due to the fact that this level is naturally the least mobile in the lumbar spine, and therefore differences in motion are small and harder to detect with a relatively small sample size. The L5-S1 level is also the most difficult to visualize accurately on a lateral radiograph due to the shadow of the sacral ala on this projection.

At the L4-L5 level, the sagittal motion data suggests that the disc replacement not only preserves motion, but can also increase or restore motion, at least in the follow-up period presented. Theoretically, by maintaining range of motion, a protective effect is imparted against future degeneration at the adjacent segments. In the future, it will be important not only to evaluate whether or not there is motion but also to qualify the type of motion that occurs across the spinal segment, as this may play a role in facet displacement and loading. Each prosthetic design will have its own motion parameters, with differing constraints and kinematics in bending, rotation, and translation. All disc replacements may maintain motion and protect the adjacent level, but the local effect at the facets may be the differentiating factor. Only long-term follow-up will reveal whether a significant effect is observed at the level adjacent to a disc replacement, and whether facet arthrosis can be prevented or will be exacerbated depending on the prosthesis design. Other issues that may exist with disc arthroplasty such as infection, wear particles, subsidence, implant failure, and longevity have not been a factor at this interim stage of the study.

Summary

In the musculoskeletal arena, low back pain is a veritable epidemic in our society today. The treatment for this common ailment, both nonoperative and operative, can often be frustrating. The current surgical standard of care, spinal fusion, is often associated with mediocre results, long recovery time, significant postoperative morbidity, and future adjacent segment degeneration. Artificial disc replacement has proven to be a promising alternative to other surgical treatments of chronic low back pain and may obviate the stigmas associated with spinal fusion. The US IDE Pivotal Clinical Trial, which has recently completed enrollment at selected clinical sites, will provide valuable information comparing this new technology to the current mainstay treatment of spinal fusion. The intermediate-term results from our site demonstrate that the objective of decreasing postoperative morbidity and improving recovery has been met. Patients who received the disc replacement as opposed to fusion had a significant improvement in pain and functional status in the early postoperative period. Over the intermediate-term, the prosthetic disc does serve to preserve motion at the surgical level(s). The more important benefit of protection of adjacent levels can only be assessed with completion of the multi-center study and long-term follow-up.

Case studies

Case 1

A 38-year-old man presented with severe back and buttock pain after discectomy at L4-5 in 1997. After the discectomy, he initially experienced some relief of his leg pain and then had progressively worsening back and buttock pain. He had a prolonged course of physical therapy, analgesic medication, and multiple epidural injections, all of which only gave him temporary mild relief. On examination, he had significant mechanical pain with flexion, extension, and side bending. Radiographs and MRI revealed moderate disc degeneration at L4-5, and minimal degeneration at L3-4 and L5-S1 (Fig. 7A, B). A discogram revealed concordant pain at L4-5 only. The patient underwent a one-level L4-5 anterior disc replacement with ProDisc-II. Clinically, the patient reported great improvement in his back pain, and was able to return to active duty as a police officer. The lateral flexion and extension radiographs on his 2-year follow-up reveal preservation of motion at L4-5 (Fig. 7C).

Case 2

A 45-year-old woman presented with intractable low back pain of at least 5 years duration. She works as a park ranger in an Alaskan national park, and her symptoms were significantly hindering her work. Her pain radiated to bilateral buttocks but no further. She had failed the gamut of nonoperative treatment, including physical therapy with multiple modalities,

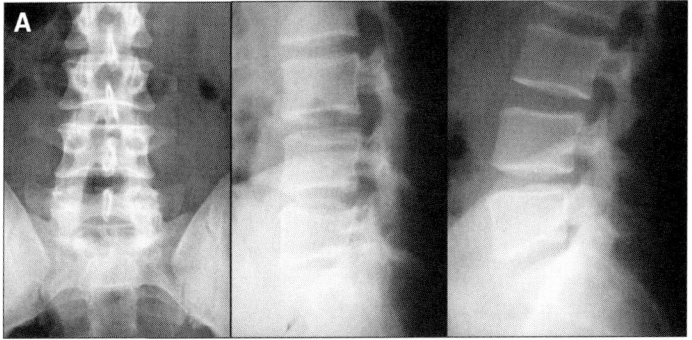
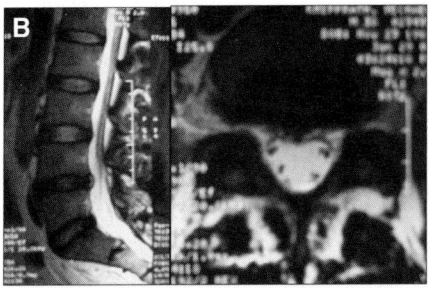
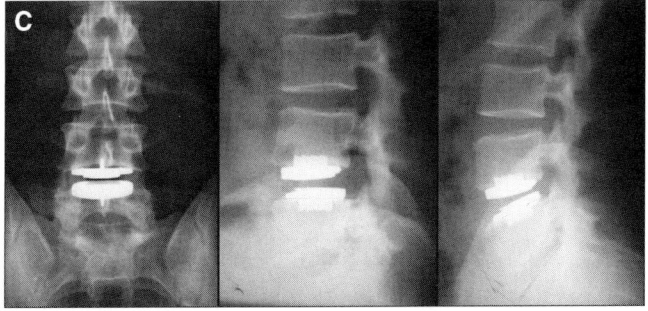

Fig. 7. Case 1 preoperative radiographs (*A*), and MRI (*B*), and postoperative anteroposterior and flexion extension radiographs (*C*).

epidural steroid injections, facet blocks, and radiofrequency ablation of her facet joint nerves. She was on Celebrex and multiple hydrocodone pills a day for pain control. Her radiographs and MRI revealed degenerated discs at L3-4 and L4-5 (Fig. 8A, B). Discograms were concordantly positive at L3-4 and L4-5. She had markedly asymmetric collapse of the disc spaces at the two affected levels, resulting in local scoliotic deformity. She successfully underwent a two-level artificial disc replacement with the ProDisc-II (Fig. 8C). By 6 months postoperatively she related outstanding pain relief and continues to do well 18 months out. She went back to work as a park ranger, was swimming, and was off all narcotic pain medications.

Case 3

A 37-year-old woman presented with an approximately 20-year history of low back pain that had been progressively deteriorating over the last several years. She denied any radiation of her pain. She was a multi-sport athlete in high school when her troubles began. She had tried exhaustive nonoperative measures for her back. She had seen chiropractors, physical therapists, taken multiple nonsteroidal anti-inflammatory pills and strong narcotic pain pills, and received acupuncture to no avail. The pain was keeping her from even her normal activities of daily living at this point. Plain radiographs revealed mild degenerative changes with anterior spurring at L3-4

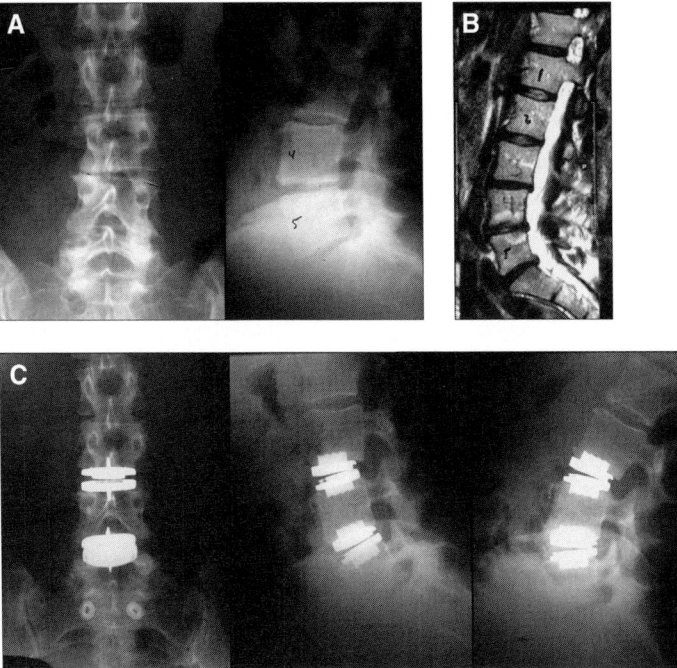

Fig. 8. Case 2 preoperative radiographs (*A*), and MRI (*B*), and postoperative anteroposterior and flexion extension radiographs (*C*). Note the dynamic correction of local scoliotic deformity at L3-5 due to asymmetric disc collapse.

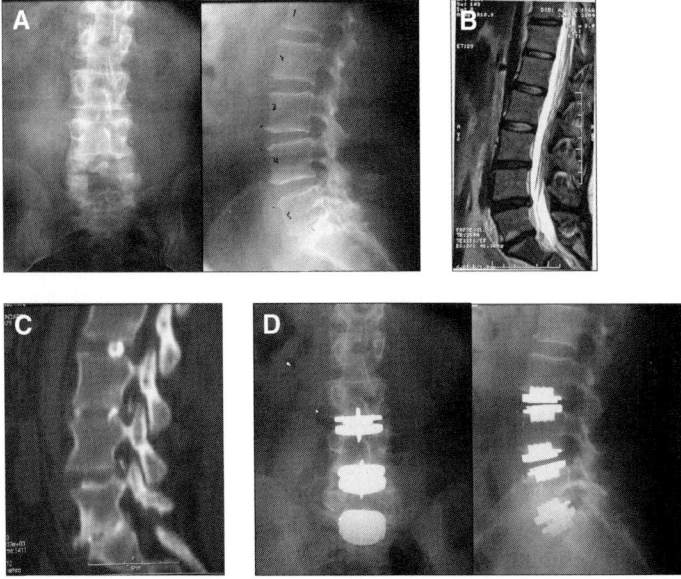

Fig. 9. Case 3 preoperative radiographs (*A*), MRI (*B*), and CT discogram (*C*), and postoperative anteroposterior and lateral radiographs (*D*).

and L4-5, but severe degenerative changes at L5-S1 with collapse of disc space (Fig. 9A). The MRI revealed desiccated discs at L3-4, L4-5, and L5-S1 (Fig. 9B). Discogram CT revealed internal disc disruption at all three levels and positive concordant pain at all three levels as well (Fig. 9C). A single or two-level fusion would not have addressed all her sources of pain and would have left a compromised disc to bear supraphysiologic loads adjacent to the lever arm of the fusion construct. Her young age also made a three-level fusion a poor surgical choice due to the risk of adjacent segment disease and her desire for an active lifestyle. Therefore a special request was made to the FDA to gain permission for the compassionate use of a three-level artificial disc replacement surgery with the ProDisc-II. This was approved and the patient successfully underwent surgery (Fig. 9D). She is approximately 6 months after surgery and doing very well. She is in an independent walking program and weaning herself off of all narcotics. She is currently on two to three hydrocodone pills a day and weaning off.

References

[1] Marnay T. Lumbar disc arthroplasty: 8–10 year results using titanium plates with a polyethylene inlay component. American Academy of Orthopaedic Surgeons annual meeting, San Francisco, CA, 2001.

[2] Marnay T. Lumbar disc replacement. Spine J 2002; 2:94S.

[3] Tropiano P, Huang RC, Girardi FP, et al. Lumbar total disc replacement. Seven to eleven-year follow-up. J Bone Joint Surg Am 2005;87-A-3:490–6.

[4] White AA, Panjabi MM. Clinical biomechanics of the spine. 2nd edition. Philadelphia (PA): JB Lippincott Co; 1990. p. 112–5.

[5] Zigler JE. ProDisc randomized multicenter trials. Total disc replacement precourse. 18th Annual Meeting of the North American Spine Society, San Diego, CA, 2003.

[6] Delamarter RB, Fribourg DM, Kanim LE, Bae H. ProDisc artificial total lumbar disc replacement: introduction and early results from the United States clinical trial. Spine 2003;28:S167–75.

[7] Bae H, Kanim L, Delamarter R. ProDisc artificial lumbar disc replacement: introduction and results from the USA clinical trial. International Society for Study of the Lumbar Spine annual meeting, Porto, Portugal, 2004.

[8] Bertagnoli R, Kumar S. Indications for full prosthetic disc arthroplasty: a correlation of clinical outcome against a variety of indications. Eur Spine J 2002; 11(Suppl 2):S131–6.

[9] Tropiano P, Huang RC, Girardi FP, Marnay T. Lumbar disc replacement: preliminary results with ProDisc II after a minimum follow-up period of 1 year. J Spinal Disord Tech 2003;16:362–8.

[10] Huang RC, Girardi FP, Cammisa Jr FP, et al. Long-term flexion-extension range of motion of the pro-disc total disc replacement. J Spinal Disord Tech 2003; 16:435–40.

[11] Cauchoix J, David T. Arthrodeses lombaires: resultats apres plus de 10 ans. Rev Chir Orthop 1985;71:263–8.

[12] Gillet P. The fate of the adjacent motion segments after lumbar fusion. J Spinal Disord 2003;16:338–45.

[13] Mayer HM, Wiechert K, Korge A, Qose I. Minimally invasive total disc replacement: surgical technique and preliminary clinical results. Eur Spine J 2002; 11(Suppl 2):S124–30.

[14] Zigler JE, Burd TA, Vialle EN, et al. Lumbar spine arthroplasty: early results using the ProDisc II: a prospective randomized trial of arthroplasty versus fusion. J Spinal Disord Tech 2003;16:352–61.

[15] Fairbank JC, Couper J, Davies JB, et al. The Oswestry low back pain disability questionnaire. Physiotherapy 1980;66:271–3.

[16] Roland M, Fairbank JC. The Roland-Morris Disability Questionnaire and the Oswestry Disability Questionnaire. Spine 2000;25:3115–24.

[17] Smith SE, Darden BV, Rhyne AL, et al. Outcome of unoperated discogram-positive low back pain. Spine 1995;20:1997–2000.

[18] Fritzell P, Hagg O, Wessberg P, et al. 2001 Volvo Award winner in clinical studies. Lumbar fusion versus nonsurgical treatment for chronic low back pain: a multicenter randomized controlled trial from the Swedish Lumbar Spine Study Group. Spine 2001;26: 2521–34.

[19] Mayer HM, Wiechert K. Microsurgical anterior approaches to the lumbar spine for interbody fusion and total disc replacement. Neurosurgery 2002; 51–5(Suppl):159–65.

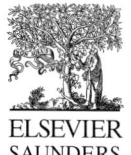

Clinical Results of Maverick Lumbar Total Disc Replacement: Two-Year Prospective Follow-up

J.C. Le Huec, MD, PhD[a],*, H. Mathews, MD[b], Y. Basso, MD[a],
S. Aunoble, MD[a], D. Hoste, MD[a], B. Bley, MD[a], T. Friesem, MD[c]

[a]*Département Orthopédie Pr Chauveaux, Spine Unit Pr Le Huec, CHU Pellegrin Tripode, Université Bordeaux 2,
Victor Segalen, 33076 Bordeaux cedex, France*
[b]*Mid-Atlantic Spine Specialists, 7650 Parham Road, Suite 200, Richmond, VA 23294-4309, USA*
[c]*University Hospital of North Tees, Nardwick, Stokton on Tees, TS 19 8PE, UK*

The development of total lumbar disk prostheses has been a logical step in the management of chronic back pain. Clinical results of studies on disk prostheses report patient satisfaction rates, Oswestry scores, and visual analog scale (VAS) assessments for back pain [1–6]; however, there has been little analysis of VAS scores for associated root pain and spine function (SF)-36 score. For example, no study has yet assessed the correlation between the clinical functional result and the position of the implants, the arthrosis of the posterior facets, or the fatty degeneration of the spinal muscles; however, such knowledge is essential for understanding the long-term outcome of devices in functional terms [7]. Disk degeneration around the device is also of prime importance because it conditions the final result in the mid- and long-term [8]. This prospective study reports the outcome of 64 Maverick (Medtronic, Memphis, Tennessee) devices implanted between January 2002 and November 2003. The minimum follow-up was 1 year, with a mean of 18 months (range, 12–36 months).

* Corresponding author.
E-mail address: j-c.lehuec@u-bordeaux2.fr
(J.C. Le Huec).

Materials and methods

Sixty-four patients were included in this prospective study, and all operations were performed by one surgeon at one center. All patients had been suffering from chronic back pain resistant to conservative treatment for at least 1 year and had received medical and rheumatologic follow-up and rehabilitation physiotherapy.

Contraindications for disk arthroplasty were the following: previous spinal surgery other than discectomy at the painful level, lumbar fracture, permanent symptomatic disk hernia, narrow lumbar canal or isthmic spondylolisthesis, scoliosis greater than 15° Cobb angle, spinal tumor, general or local infection, evolving autoimmune disease, pregnancy, morbid obesity, psychiatric disturbances, and major bone disease.

Inclusion criteria were as follows: age between 20 and 60 years irrespective of sex, symptomatic degenerative lumbar discopathy as evidenced by radiography and MRI, failure of conservative treatment given for longer than 12 months, Oswestry score >30%, predominant chronic back pain, and absence of permanent nerve root compression.

The 64 patients had a mean age of 44 years (SD 7), a mean height of 1.68 m (SD 0.09), and a mean weight of 68 kg (SD 12). There were 39 women and 25 men, all Caucasian. Thirty percent were smokers and 9% had back pain associated with a work accident. Professionally, 20 were attending work, 21 were absent because of their back pain, and 23 were no longer able to work. Eighteen patients underwent previous spinal treatment including three isolated rhyzolyses of the posterior facets and four disk annuloplasties by radiofrequency at the painful level (one of which was followed by discectomy). Eight patients had received disk nucleolysis with chemopapain (one of which was followed by discectomy). Twenty-four patients had a history of abdominal surgery as follows: 13 appendectomies, 2 extrauterine pregnancies, 6 cesarean sections, 3 surgeries for groin hernia, 2 cholecystectomies, 4 tubal ligations under celioscopy, and 2 hysterectomies.

Levels to be operated were the following: L5-S1 disc prosthesis (35 cases), L4-L5 disc prosthesis (14 cases), L5-S1 arthrodesis with L4-L5 disc prosthesis (13 cases), and L3-L4 disc prosthesis (2 cases).

All patients had received radiologic, static, dynamic, and load-bearing evaluations in addition to MRI. Preoperataive MRI was used to assess the state of the disk. Disk degeneration was measured on T2-weighted sagittal slices and classified as described by Fujiwara et al [8]: grade 1, normal disk; grade 2, normal height with median transversal dark band; grade 3, normal height but with hypointensity; grade 4, slightly decreased height accompanied by inhomogeneous hypointensity; and grade 5, clearly diminished hypointense heterogeneous disk with hyperintense transversal lines. High intensity zones were noted. For facet arthrosis, the MRI classification described by Fujiwara et al [9] was used: grade 1, normal facets; grade 2, moderately compressed facets with small osteophytes; grade 3, facets with subchondral sclerosis and moderate osteophytes; and grade 4, facets lacking articular joint space and with large osteophytes. For muscle degeneration, Goutallier et al's [10] scale was applied: grade 1, normal muscle; grade 2, muscle interspersed with some fat; grade 3, as much muscle as fat; and grade 4, more fat than muscle.

Radiography was used to examine mobility during flexion–extension around the device and at the two adjacent levels. Sagittal equilibrium was assessed by radiography in the standing anteroposterior (AP) and lateral positions. Measurements performed by an independent radiologist on AP and lateral radiographs were accurate to 3° for angles and 3 mm for distances. Implant position was defined according to coronal radiographs as shown in Fig. 1. In this way, the keel of the device serves as a landmark to establish its position. The symmetric center of the vertebra corresponds coronally to the midpoint of its width. The distance between the midpoint of the vertebra and the keel of the device is related to the radius of the vertebra and expressed as a percentage. When the device is centered, its degree of lateralization is 0%. The more lateralized it is, the closer it is to a score of 100%. The authors' arbitrary rating system is as follows: 0% to 9%, well centered; 1% to 19%,

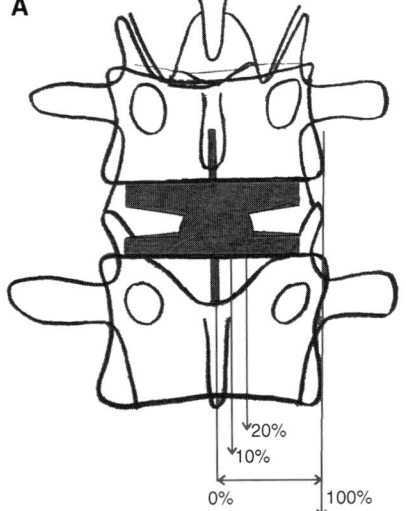
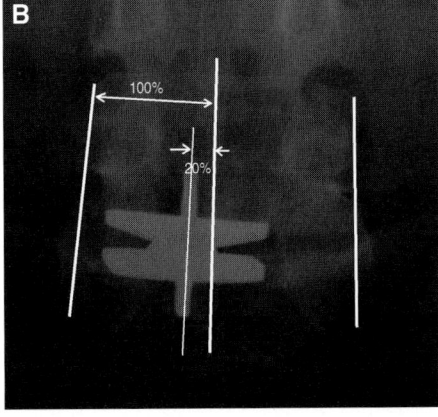

Fig. 1. Implant position on anteroposterior radiographic view. The distance between midpoint of the vertebra and the keel of the device is related to the radius of the vertebra and expressed as a percentage. (*A*) Position of the keel is calculated on anteroposterior view; 0%, 10%, 20% define the position in the series. (*B*) Example of the worst implant position.

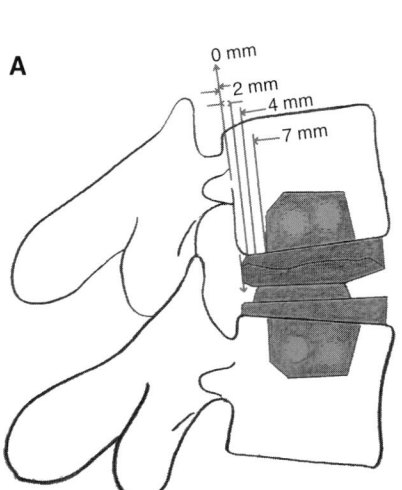
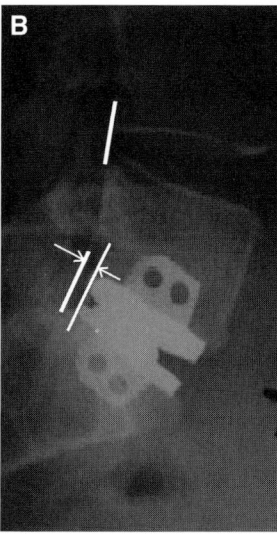

Fig. 2. Implant position on a lateral radiographic view. (*A*) Position of the prosthesis is calculated on lateral view according to the distance between posterior edge of the implant and posterior edge of the inferior vertebra. (*B*) Example of prosthesis position in group 4–7 mm.

moderately off center; 20% and above, off center. Implant position was defined on lateral radiographs as shown in Fig. 2. The position of the device was defined according to the distance between its posterior edge and the posterior edge of the inferior vertebral body of the segment. To obtain a value independent from the radiographic enlargement factor, measurements were related to the size of the keel of the device, which was constant whatever the model. If the device was too posterior (in the vertebral canal), the distance was expressed as a negative value. A distance from the posterior edge of the vertebra between 4 and 7 mm was considered to represent a moderately correct position, whereas a distance <4 mm was taken to be satisfactory. Any distance >7 mm was considered inadequate (see Fig. 2).

The prosthesis is inserted by a mini-invasive anterior approach [11], with complete discectomy and release of the discal space. The patient is positioned supine in the so-called "French position," with legs bent and open laterally [12,13]. The surgeon stands between the legs facing the lumbar spine in the cephalad-caudal direction, which is ergonomic for checking the midline of the spine when approaching the L5-S1 and L4-L5 levels. The assistant stands on the right or left side of the patient. The incision is longitudinal or horizontal crossing the midline and 7 to 8 cm long. A Pfannenstiel incision is more cosmetic for one-level surgery. After vertical incision of the rectus abdominis sheath, the muscle is retracted laterally to reach the common fascia of the external oblique muscle. The retroperitoneal space is reached and the peritoneal sac retracted. The peritoneal sac is pushed to the contralateral side with the ureter and the hypogastric plexus. The vessel bifurcation is now exposed and analyzed. To reach L5-S1, the left iliac vein must be carefully retracted and the medial sacral vessels ligated. An opening to the anterior part of the L5-S1 disc of least 32 mm must be exposed. At the L4-L5 level, the left approach is commonly used. The surgeon must pay attention to the ascending lumbar vein, which is located at the corner of the psoas belly and the left iliac vein. This important collateral must be ligated. The segmental vessels at L4 and L5 must also be ligated to allow retraction of the aorta and vena cava. Traction on the left iliac vein must be controlled throughout the procedure. The anterior part of the disc is opened according to the size of the templates. The anterior anulus and nucleus are removed using disc rongeur, kerisson, curettes, and a scraper. The posterior anulus must be opened to free the disc space and to allow good restoration of the disc height. It is not necessary to open the posterior longitudinal ligament, but it must be detached from the posterior border of the end plates using the specific instruments. The mobility of the disc space is tested with a spreader under C-arm control. The midline is checked with AP fluoroscopy. A dedicated instrument is introduced in the disc space and makes it possible to create a parallel distraction of the disc, thus restoring the disk height. The upper or the lower keel cutter is slid onto a guide and impacted into

Table 1
Mean Oswestry score and leg and back pain visual analog scale scores at each follow-up

Score	Preoperative	1 mo	3 mo	6 mo	1 y	2 y
Oswestry	43.8	34.8*	26.3*	24.2*	22.8*	23.1*
Leg Pain	3.9	3	2.7	2*	2.4*	2.1*
Back Pain	7.6	3.7*	3*	3*	3.5*	3.2*

* $P < 0.05$.

the vertebral body to prepare the bed for the fin of the prosthesis. The prosthesis is impacted into the prepared disc space under fluoroscopic control. The retractors are carefully removed and bleeding is controlled. The rectus abdominis fascia and subcutaneous fat are closed with drainage.

The implant (Maverick) is a metal-on-metal disc prosthesis made of cobalt-chrome, with a ball-and-socket design. The prosthesis has a fixed posterior center of rotation located below the lower end plate. The production of wear debris is low and without epidural reaction on animal studies [3,12,14].

All patients were seen postoperatively at 1, 3, and 6 months and at 1 and 2 years. Pain was assessed using a VAS, neurologic function, Oswestry scores, and the SF-36 [15]. Clinical success was taken to be a 25% improvement on the Oswestry score (ie, the success rate defined by the US Food and Drug Administration [FDA] in a randomized prospective study concerning the SB Charité prosthesis) [16]. Degree of patient satisfaction was noted, as were need of analgesics and duration of treatment with analgesics or anti-inflammatory agents. All patients received postoperative physiotherapy from 1 week post surgery and wore a supple girdle for 6 weeks. Statistical analysis was with the Student t test and the χ^2 test.

Results

All patients underwent follow-up examinations. Oswestry score preoperatively and at 2 years' follow-up was 43.8 and 23.1, respectively. Low back pain improved from a mean VAS of 7.6 ± 1.7 preoperatively to 3.2 ± 1.8 at 2 years. Mean leg pain VAS score decreased from 3.9 preoperatively to 2.1 at 2 years ($P < 0.05$). Mean daily duration of back pain decreased from 70% to 40% ($P < 0.05$). Daily duration of leg pain decreased from 36% to 20% ($P < 0.05$). According to the FDA criteria (>25% improvement of Oswestry score) [17], the success rate was 75% ($P < 0.05$). Improvement in back pain directly affected the improvement in Oswestry score ($P = 0.008$) (Table 1).

Evolution of SF-36 score was weighted according to sex and age of the patient. An improvement greater than 15% was considered a success [7,16]. Thus, 85% of patients experienced physical improvement at 1 year, whereas improvement of mental health was noted in 43%.

The mean hospital stay was 4.6 days (range, 3–10 days).

Complications

There were 4 cases of postoperative root pain and 2 cases with sequelae from previous surgery (discectomies). Seventeen patients received posterior facet infiltration (11 with a good result). Three patients had spinal pain other than in the lumbar region. One patient had a superficial infection treated by local debridement. There was one visceral lesion due to the surgical incision, which was damage to a ureter in a female patient operated several times for gynecologic problems. The damage was successfully repaired and the orthopedic result was excellent. Minor intraoperative complications were noted due to the surgical approach in 11 cases. There was never any breakage of the device. No implant had to be removed or surgically revised.

Table 2
Prosthesis motion at the operated level

	Prosthesis motion at disc L5-S1	Prosthesis motion at disc L4-L5	Prosthesis motion at disc L4-L5 with L5-S1 arthrodesis	Prosthesis at disc L3-L4
n	35	14	13	2
Average	7.9	9.4	7.4	7.1

Table 3
Position of the prosthesis on anteroposterior radiograph

	Well centered	Moderately off center	Off center
Degree of Lateralization	0%–9%	10%–19%	>19%
n	51	13	0
Average	2.80%	17.40%	0%

Consumption of analgesics was reduced overall because no patient needed any morphine-based drugs postoperatively, whereas 62% were taking them preoperatively. With regard to resumption of professional activity, 63% returned to work (the mean time to return to work was 5 months; range, 2 months to 1 year). When the Oswestry score was improved by 25% or more, there was a 44.4% chance of returning to work. When the score improved 75%, the chance of returning to work was 73% ($P = 0.004$). Factors influencing the clinical result in terms of success were as follows: young age was associated with a good result ($P = 0.05$) and female sex was associated with better results ($P = 0.003$). Alternatively, previous spine surgery decreased the chance of having a good result ($P = 0.005$), whereas being off work before the intervention did not influence clinical outcome ($P = 0.14$).

Radiologic results

Mobility in flexion and extension was 7.9° at discs L5-S1, 9.4° at L4-L5, and 7.4° at L4-L5 when there was an arthrodesis at L5-S1 (Table 2). The coronal position of the device was considered excellent in 51 cases (79.6%) and satisfactory in 13 cases (20.4%); there was no insertion with an offset superior to 19% (Table 3). The position of the implant on lateral radiography was considered excellent in 57 cases (89%) and satisfactory in 7 cases (11%) (Table 4). No implant was inserted with a distance superior to 7 mm from the posterior wall of the inferior vertebra. There was no correlation between

Table 4
Position of the prosthesis on lateral radiograph

	Satisfactory	Moderately correct	Inadequate
Distance	0–4 mm	4–7 mm	>7 mm
n	57	7	0
Average	1.07	5.1	0

Distance was measured from posterior edge of vertebrae.

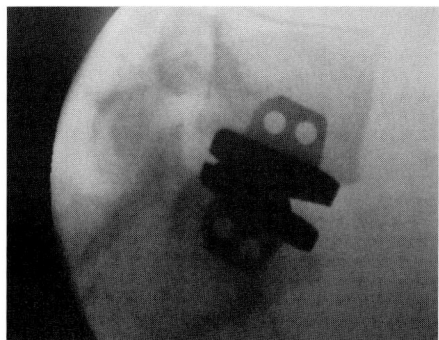

Fig. 3. Posterior subsidence of the implant: 4 mm stable over time, with excellent clinical outcome.

satisfactory functional outcome (Oswestry >25% and VAS >2 improvement) and the position of the device based on the criteria applied in AP and lateral radiographs.

Postoperatively, the device migrated axially 3 to 5 mm in the region of the superior end plate in five patients (Fig. 3). Subsidence was stable at 1-year follow-up. The outcome was satisfactory in three of these patients, with an Oswestry score averaging 14 and a VAS pain score of 2. For the other two patients, one had a very poor result (Oswestry improvement zero) and the other had a poor result (Oswestry improvement 10). There was no case of anterior or posterior migration. Three patients had heterotopic ossification (two type 1, one type 3 according to McAfee classification) [17]; all were mobile on dynamic radiographs.

Correlations between improvement in Oswestry score and radiologically diagnosed criteria were as follows: facet osteoarthritis grade 1 or 2 did not influence outcome ($P = 0.82$); the presence of high intensity zones in the indication did not influence outcome ($P = 0.66$); the presence of an osteophyte did not influence outcome ($P = 0.69$); the presence of intradiscal gas did not influence outcome ($P = 0.34$); and the presence of a change in Modic-type 1 or 2 signal in the indication did not influence outcome ($P = 0.33$).

Alternatively, certain criteria influenced functional outcome: muscle degeneration grades 1 and 2 led to a better outcome than grades 3 and 4 ($P = 0.006$); and absence of McNab osteophytes on the spine other than at the operated region were associated with success ($P = 0.003$).

The position of the implant on AP radiographs did not influence outcome when the implant was situated between 0% and 19% ($P < 0.05$). The position of the implant on lateral view radiographs did not influence outcome when the implant was situated between 0 and 7 mm from the posterior wall of the inferior vertebra ($P < 0.05$).

Discussion

Discectomy with insertion of total disk prosthesis has been widely reported to improve the clinical symptoms of chronic back pain [5,6,16,18–20]. The degree of improvement is equivalent to that obtained with anterior fusion cages using the mini-invasive technique [21]. Radiographic follow-up in the authors' series showed a degree of mobility close to normal [14,22] and confirms the results obtained with other devices such as the SB Charité (Depuy, USA), as reported by many authors [5,6,16,17,19,20], and with the Prodisc (Synthes, Switzerland), as reported by Bertagnoli and Kumar [2] and Mayer et al [11]. The technique is safe because the intra- and postoperative complication rate is low and equivalent to other series [2,3,16]. The patients recover rapidly, and the mean hospital stay of 3 to 5 days is similar to the results reported by Bertagnoli and Kumar [2] and Lemaire et al [5] but in contrast to 8 to 12 days for an arthrodesis reported by Katz [23]. The Oswestry score improved for 75% of patients; this improvement is significantly correlated with facet arthrosis and fatty muscle degeneration. It has been demonstrated that the disc degenerates before the facets [24], but facet arthrosis could be a limiting factor for total disc replacement, particularly in adjacent level disease after fusion [25,26]. This study is the first to show that a semiconstrained implant with a fixed posterior center of rotation can be implanted with grade 1 and 2 facet arthrosis with a good clinical outcome. This result seems to confirm the work of Dooris et al [27] showing that a posterior center of rotation lightens the load on the facets. This study is also the first to show a relationship between muscle fatty degeneration and clinical results because the greater the amount of fat, the less satisfactory the result. Contrary to the posterior approach, the anterior implantation technique does not damage the spinal muscles and shortens the delay until activity can be resumed.

The SF-36 physical score improved more than the mental score, similar to the prospective randomized study results using the SB Charité device [16].

The position of the implant on AP and lateral radiographs was satisfactory with the instruments used; all were implanted in good or excellent position. The functional outcome (Oswestry and VAS scores) did not correlate with the implant position when the device was implanted in a safety region demarcated on coronal and lateral views, respectively, as defined in the protocol. Outside this safe area, the results could be different; however, there were no data to confirm this.

In summary, a semiconstrained device with a fixed center of rotation is a biomechanical tradeoff for obtaining a very good clinical outcome, providing the device is implanted within the safety margins previously outlined. This report is the first to show such an outcome. Other disc prosthesis designs were less successful in the past [18,28,29].

Disc prostheses offer the prospect of earlier treatment of certain recalcitrant chronic back pain without having recourse to an arthrodesis. It is always possible to revert to an arthrodesis if results are poor or if there is progressive degeneration of the posterior structures [25]. A few cases of arthrodesis with posterior fixation and a posterolateral graft have been reported by Lemaire et al [5] for treating patients whose pain is recalcitrant. The failure may be due to a technical error or to an erroneous indication, so patients should be selected according to very rigorous criteria. Le Huec et al [12] proposed guidelines that take into account the characteristics of not only the pathologic level (disk and posterior elements) but also the adjacent levels. The spontaneous fusion of certain prostheses has been reported by Lemaire et al [5], a problem always accompanied by intraprosthetic calcification. One solution is to prescribe postoperative nonsteroidal anti-inflammatory drugs, as in hip prostheses. Another solution is to limit the bleeding of the vertebral end plates by applying a hemostatic agent on the bony tissue not covered by the prosthesis. Even heterotopic calcifications allowed the prosthesis to be mobile in three of the authors' cases. Based on the McAfee classification [17], it is not possible to know whether these patients will reach grade 4 calcification and, therefore, lose their mobility. The metal-on-metal couple seems very safe as demonstrated by animal studies [14] and previous work in total hip replacement by Jacobs et al [30] and Haynes et al [31]. The quantity of wear debris produced by a metal-on-metal implant is low compared with metal-on-polyethylene prostheses [30]. Le Huec et al [32] showed that there was no shock absorption difference between metal-on-metal and metal-on-polyethylene disc prostheses in physiologic conditions. Prosthesis dislocation has been reported for Prodisc [33] and SB Charité prostheses [34] but not with the Maverick implant. The design of the Maverick in respect to fundamental criteria proposed

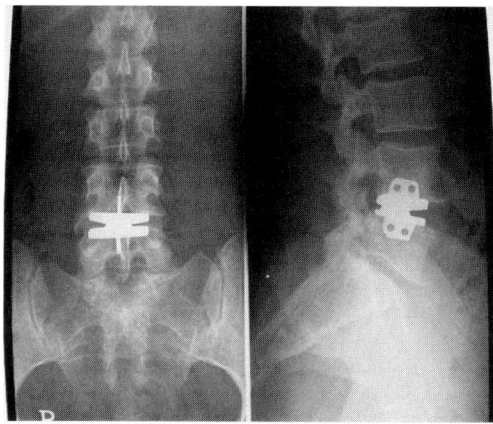

Fig. 4. Excellent position on anteroposterior and lateral views with excellent clinical outcome.

by Hedman et al [35] and Dooris [27] is likely very important regarding the biomechanics.

Summary

The metal-on-metal Maverick device with a posterior center of rotation and controlled translation is a promising therapeutic technique (Fig. 4). Its mechanical characteristics and resistance to wear make it an interesting option in terms of its life cycle. Only long-term follow-up exceeding 5 years will make it possible to confirm these favorable preliminary results and to analyze the effects on the segments adjacent to the operated levels. This series shows that for one-level degenerative disc disease, the early results are equivalent to the best anterior lumbar interbody fusion series [21], with a low complication rate. Total disc replacement could offer benefit by preventing adjacent-level disease because of decreased stress on the adjacent disc after the sagittal balance is restored [36].

References

[1] Allen MJ, Myer BJ, Millet PJ, et al. The effects of particulate cobalt, chromium, and cobalt-chromium alloy on human osteoblast-like cells in vitro. J Bone Joint Surg Br 1997;79:475–82.

[2] Bertagnoli R, Kumar S. Indications for full prosthetic disc arthroplasty: a correlation of clinical out-come against a variety of indications. Eur Spine J 2002; 11(2):131–6.

[3] Cinotti G, David T, Postacchini F. Results of disc prosthesis after a minimum follow-up period of 2 years. Spine 1996;21:995–1000.

[4] Enker P, Steffee A, McMillin C, et al. Artificial disc replacement: preliminary report with a 3-year minimum follow-up. Spine 1993;18:1061–70.

[5] Lemaire JP, Skalli W, Lavaste F, et al. Intervertebral disc prosthesis: results and prospects for the year 2000. Clin Orthop 1997;337:64–76.

[6] Zeegers WS, Bohnen LMU, Laaper M, et al. Artificial disc replacement with the modular type SB Charité III: 2-year results in 50 prospectively studied patients. Eur Spine J 1999;8:210–7.

[7] Mayer HM, Korge A. Non fusion technology in degenerative lumbar spinal disorders: facts, questions, challenges. Eur Spine J 2002;11(2):85–91.

[8] Fujiwara A, Tamai K, An HS, et al. The relationship between disc degeneration, facet joint osteoarthritis, and stability of the degenerative lumbar spine. J Spinal Disord 2000;13(5):444–50.

[9] Fujiwara A, Tamai K, An HS, et al. Orientation and osteoarthritis of the lumbar facet joint. Clin Orthop 2001;385:88–94.

[10] Goutallier D, Postel JM, Bernageau J, et al. Fatty muscle degeneration in cuff ruptures. Pre- and postoperative evaluation by CT scan. Clin Orthop 1994; 304:78–83.

[11] Mayer HM, Wiechert K, Korge A, et al. Minimally invasive total disc replacement: surgical technique and preliminary results. Eur Spine J 2002;11(2):124–30.

[12] Le Huec JC, Aunoble S, Friesem T, et al. Maverick total lumbar disk prosthesis: biomechanics and preliminary clinical results. In: Gunzburg R, Spalzski M, editors. Arthroplasty of the spine. Lippincott; 2004. p. 53–8.

[13] Le Huec JC, Aunoble S, Magendie J, et al. Video-assisted anterior approach to the spine. In: Duparc J, editor. Surgical techniques in orthopaedics and traumatology. Editions scientifiques et médicales. Paris: Elsevier SAS; 2003. p. 55–;060-D-I0.

[14] Mathews Hallett H, Le Huec JC, Friesem T, et al. Design rationale and biomechanics of Maverick total disc arthroplasty with early clinical results. Spine J 2004;4(61001):S268–75.

[15] Frymoyer JW. Indications for consideration of the artificial disco. In: Weinstein JN, editor. Clinical efficacy and outcome in the diagnosis and treatment of low back pain. New York: Raven Press; 1992. p. 227–36.

[16] Guyer RD, McAfee PC, Hochschuler SH, et al. Prospective randomized study of the Charité artificial disc: data from two investigational centers. Spine J 2004;4(Suppl 6):S252–9.

[17] McAfee PC, Cunningham BW, Devine J, et al. Classification of heterotopic ossification (HO) in artificial disk replacement. J Spinal Disord Tech 2003;16(4): 384–9.

[18] Cunningham BW, Lowery GL, Serhan HA, et al. Total disc replacement arthroplasty using the acroflex lumbar disc: a non human primate model. Eur Spine J 2002;11(2):115–23.

[19] Griffith SL, Shelokov AP, Buttner-Janz K, et al. A multicenter retrospective study of the clinical results of the LINK SB Charité intervertebral prosthesis: the initial European experience. Spine 1994;19:1842–9.

[20] Hochschuler SR, Ohnmeiss DD, Guyer RD, et al. Artificial disc: preliminary results of a prospective study in the United States. Eur Spine J 2002;11(2): 106–10.

[21] Burkus JK, Gornet MF, Dickman CA, et al. Anterior lumbar interbody fusion using rhBMP-2 with tapered interbody cages. J Spinal Disord Tech 2002;15(5): 337–49.

[22] Buttner-Janz K, Schellnack K, Zippel H. Biomechanics of the SB Charité lumbar intervertebral disc endoprosthesis. Int Orthop 1989;13:173–6.

[23] Katz JN. Lumbar spinal fusion: surgical rates, costs, and complications. Spine 1995;20(Suppl):78–83.

[24] Butler D, Trafimow JH, Andersson GB, et al. Discs degenerate before facets. Spine 1990;15:111–3.

[25] Eck JC, Humphreys SC, Hodges SD. Adjacent-segment degeneration after lumbar fusion: a review of clinical, biomechanical, and radiologic studies. Am J Orthop 1999;28:336–40.

[26] Lee CK. Accelerated degeneration of the segment adjacent to a lumbar fusion. Spine 1988;13:375–7.

[27] Dooris AP, Goel VK, Grosland NM, et al. Load sharing between anterior and posterior elements in a lumbar motion segment implanted with an artificial disc. Spine 2001;26:122–9.

[28] Ferstrom U. Arthroplasty with intercorporal endoprosthesis in herniated disc and painful disc. Acta Orthop Scand 1996;10(IJ):287–9.

[29] Kostuik JP. Intervertebral disc replacement: experimental study. Clin Orthop 1997;337:27–41.

[30] Jacobs IL, Skipor AK, Doorn PF, et al. Cobalt and chromium concentrations in patients with metal on metal total hip replacements. Clin Orthop 1996; 329(Suppl):256–63.

[31] Haynes D, Rogers S, Hay S, et al. The differences in toxicity and release of bone resorbing mediators induced by titanium and cobalt-chromium alloy wear particles. J Bone Joint Surg Am 1993;75(6): 825–34.

[32] Le Huec JC, Kiaer T, Friesem T, et al. Shock absorption in lumbar disc prosthesis, a preliminary mechanical study. J Spinal Disord 2003;16:346–51.

[33] Aunoble S, Donkersloot P, Le Huec JC. Dislocations with intervertebral disc prosthesis: two case reports. Eur Spine J 2004;13:464–7.

[34] Van Ooij A. Complications of artificial disk replacement: a report of 27 patients with SB Charité disc. J Spinal Disord Tech 2003;4:369–83.

[35] Hedman TP, Kostuik JP, Fernie GR, et al. Design of an intervertebral disc prosthesis. Spine 1991;16:256–60.

[36] Le Huec JC, Basso Y, Mathews H, et al. The effect of single level total disc arthroplasty on sagittal balance parameters: a prospective study. Eur Spine J 2005, in press.

Clinical Results of Charité Lumbar Total Disc Replacement

John J. Regan, MD[a,b],*

[a]Institute for Spinal Disorders, Cedars-Sinai Medical Center, Los Angeles, CA 90048, USA
[b]California Spine Group, 120 S. Spalding Drive, Suite 400, Beverly Hills, CA 90212, USA

In an effort to preserve segmental lumbar motion and to prevent adjacent segment disease, there has been a growing enthusiasm for the use of intervertebral disc prosthesis as an alternative to segmental lumbar fusion. To date, more than 100-disc prostheses have been designed, but only 10 prostheses have been approved and implanted in humans. The Charité Artificial Disc has had the longest clinical follow-up with more than 5000 implantations in over 30 countries and reported >10-year satisfactory results [1–7].

The development of the SB Charité prosthesis began in the early 1980s by Kurt Schellnack and Karin Büttner-Janz at Charité Hospital in Berlin, Germany. The artificial disc prosthesis was designed as an unconstrained three-component implant made from two metal endplates with an interposed polyethylene-sliding core. Since the world's first human implantation in 1984, three generations of the lumbar SB Charité prosthesis have been introduced. In Type I SB Charité, the endplates were stainless steel, 1 mm thick, and round. Initially, 11 fixation teeth, each 2 mm long, were used at the periphery, which was later revised to three anterior and two posterior teeth. These implants, placed in 13 patients, were complicated by subsidence into the vertebral body due to high concentrated stress in the small surface area of contact between the metal endplate and the vertebra. This led to enlargement of the endplates with the Type II SB Charité and placement of 44 implants in 36 patients (1985–1987). However, Type II implants experienced high rates of fatigue failure at the junction of the lateral wing and the center of the implant. This failure was attributed to the implant material (nonforged stainless steel) and the lack of congruity between the vertebral endplate and the metal endplate. Type I and Type II SB Charité were implanted in total of 49 patients at the Charité Hospital. In 1987, Waldemar LINK GmbH & Co revised the endplate design and material and manufactured the Type III SB Charité or the LINK SB Charité in Hamburg, Germany (Figs. 1, 2). The implant has recently adopted a new name, Charité Artificial Disc, after it was purchased by DePuy Spine (Johnson & Johnson, Raynham, MA). The endplates are made of cobalt-chrome-molybdenum (CoCrMo) alloy with a convexity to better match the concavity of the vertebral endplates. A bioactive coating, TiCaP, for bony on-growth has been available worldwide since 1998 except in the United States. The unconstrained sliding-core is a bi-convex polyethylene that is interposed between the inner concavities of the endplates with a radiopaque wire for radiographic visualization. Endplate fixation is obtained with three fixation teeth anteriorly and three posteriorly, each measuring 2.5 mm in height. Currently, five implant sizes (1 through 5), four sliding core sizes (7.5, 8.5, 9.5, 10.5, 11.5), and oblique endplates (0°, 5°, 7.5°, 10°) are available to allow a variety of surgical options in restoring segmental lordosis and to achieve parallel alignment of the inner metal endplates.

Spine biomechanics and artificial disc replacement

Lumbar spine involves very complex kinematics with an intricate interplay between the disc, posterior facets, and ligaments. White and Panjabi as well as other investigators [8,9] have extensively studied the

* Institute for Spinal Disorders, Cedars-Sinai Hospital, Los Angeles, CA 90048.
E-mail address: jjregan@spinesource.com

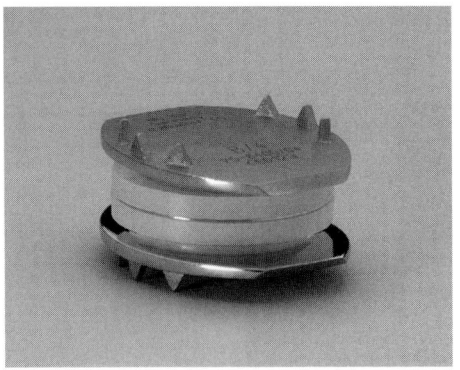

Fig. 1. Charité artificial disc. (*Courtesy of* DePuy Spine, Raynham, MA; with permission.)

characteristics of lumbar motion and have defined segmental range of motion, coupling patterns, and Instant Axis of Rotation (IAR). The position of the IAR has been described as not being a constant point and moving posteriorly with extension and anteriorly with flexion. Anterior translation of the cephalad vertebrae is coupled with flexion, which is an important element of segmental lumbar motion as it removes stress from the posterior facet joints [5]. The Charité Artificial Disc was designed to recreate the physiologic coupling pattern as well as the variable IAR of the lumbar spine [5,10]. The floating sliding core of the unconstrained three-component prosthesis replicates the physiologic coupling action as it translates anteriorly with flexion and posteriorly with extension. An accurate prosthesis placement, within 0–3 mm posterior to the midline of the vertebral body, is required to simulate the lumbar kinematics as described by White and Panjabi [9].

Indications

As with any other surgical intervention, patient selection and proper indication is the most important factor in predicting good surgical outcome. Unlike degenerated peripheral joints in which pain is generated as a result of movement of two destroyed cartilaginous surfaces, pain generator in lumbar degenerative disease is more complex and less understood. Only patients with pure discogenic back pain secondary to degenerative disc disease are candidates for lumbar total disc replacement. Therefore, it is critical to obtain a detailed clinical history, physical examination, and adequate imaging studies

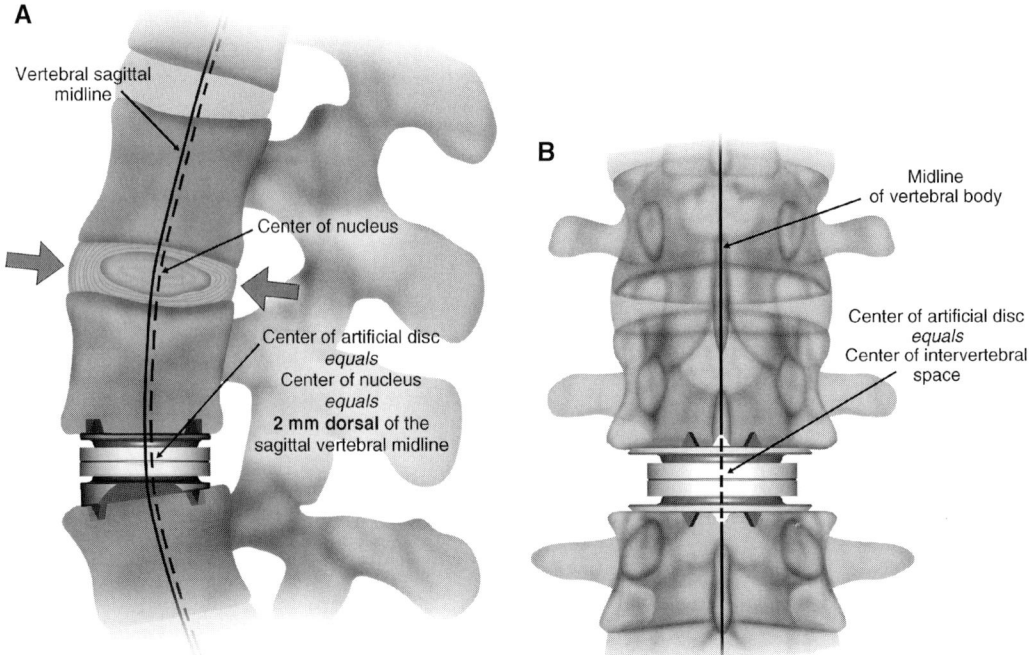

Fig. 2. (*A*) Ideal position of implant on lateral view 2mm behind mid-sagittal plane. (*B*) Ideal midline position of prosthesis in anteroposterior view. (*Courtesy of* DePuy Spine, Raynham, MA; with permission.)

to diagnose discogenic back pain and to use diagnostic provocative discography to confirm this entity if needed. Posterior facets should be carefully evaluated on physical exam and on the imaging studies such as MRI and CT scans. If posterior facet disease is suspected, diagnostic injection may be used to rule out this condition as the contributing source of pain as theses patients do not benefit from total disc replacement. The following outline of indication and contraindications was set forth by the US Investigational Device Exemption (IDE) trial for the Charité Artificial Disc, which was initiated in 2000. The randomized study with 2-year follow-up is now complete. Currently, multiple-level Charité implantation is only performed outside of US.

Age 18–60 years
Single-level disease at L4/L5 or L5/S1
Symptomatic Degenerative Disc Disease (DDD) with objective evidence of lumbar DDD by CT or MRI. Provocative discogram may also be used as a confirmatory test. Degenerative disc disease is defined as discogenic back pain with degeneration of the disc as confirmed by history and radiographic studies with one or more of the following:
Contained herniated nucleus pulposus
Paucity of facet joint degeneration
Decrease of intervertebral disc height of at least 4 mm
Scarring/thickening of the annulus fibrosis with osteophytes indicating osteoarthritis
Leg pain or back pain in the absence of nerve root compression as determined by MRI or CT scan, without prolapse or narrowing of lateral recess
At least 6 months of failed conservative management

Contraindications

Previous thoracic or lumbar fusion
Previous spine surgery at the affected level except prior discectomy, nondestabilizing laminectomy/otomy without facetectomy, or nucleolysis
Osteoporosis or metabolic bone disease. Osteoporosis is defined as bone mineral density of more than 1 standard deviation below the norm for matched age group
Single or bilateral radicular leg pain on straight leg test (pain radiating past the knee into lower extremity) in the presence of a documented disc herniation.
Lumbar scoliosis (>11 degrees of coronal deformity)
Mid-sagittal stenosis of <8 mm, as measured by CT or MRI
Lateral recess stenosis
Segmental instability defined as more than 3 mm of motion in flexion and extension
Spondylolysis
Spondylolisthesis >3mm
Lumbar spinal stenosis, central and lateral recess
Morbid obesity (body mass index over 40% or more than 100 lbs over ideal body weight)
Spinal neoplasm
Active systemic or local infection
Facet joint arthrosis.
Pregnancy
History of chronic steroid use
Arachnoiditis
Metal allergy
Autoimmune disorders
Psychosocial disorder (Waddel score >3)
Previous retro-peritoneal or >3 intra-abdominal operations

Case examples

Case 1. A 28-year-old disabled actor presented with intractable low back pain recalcitrant to 2 years of nonoperative management including anti-inflammatory medications, physical therapy, acupuncture, and steroid injections. He complained of morning stiffness and pain, especially with changing posture and minimal bilateral buttocks pain. Patient reported an Oswestry Disability Index (ODI) of 85 and Visual Analog Scale (VAS) of 8. MRI scan of the lumbar spine revealed degenerated and collapsed disc space at L5-S1. Provocative discogram revealed a positive concordant pain with relief after infusion of anesthetics. He was diagnosed with discogenic low back pain based on his history, MRI, and confirmatory provocative discography. MRI axial views of the L5-S1 revealed normal morphology of the posterior facets without any degeneration. This patient was thought to be an ideal candidate for total disc replacement as it would preserve segmental motion and potentially decrease the risk of adjacent segment disease. After an uncomplicated surgery, patient's ODI and VAS score decreased to 20 and 3 at 6 weeks, respectively, and maintained at 2 years of follow-up (Figs. 3, 4).

Case 2. A 35-year-old man referred to our institution for evaluation as a potential candidate for lumbar total disc replacement. He complained of worsening low back pain with associated bilateral leg

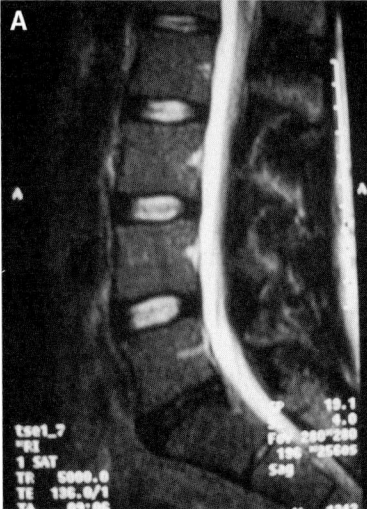
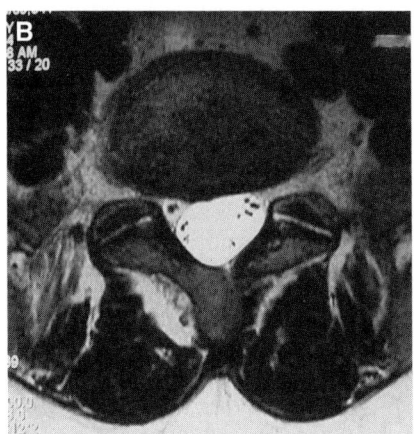

Fig. 3. (*A*, *B*) Lateral and axial view of MRI with disc degeneration at L5-S1.

pain for the past 3 years and failed nonoperative management. Lumbar radiographs and MRI revealed degenerative disc disease at L5-S1 with normal adjacent levels. However, there was also evidence of pars fracture with grade I spondylolisthesis at L5-S1 that was confirmed with a CT scan. Lumbar TDR was not offered to this patient as pars fracture with spondylolisthesis is a contraindication to this operation as it would render the operated segment unstable. He underwent an uncomplicated lumbar interbody fusion and decompression with significant improvement of his symptoms (Fig. 5).

Preoperative planning

Access surgeon

Typically an experienced vascular or a general surgeon performs the retroperitoneal approach at

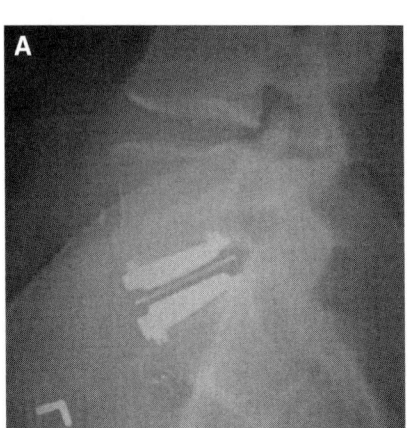
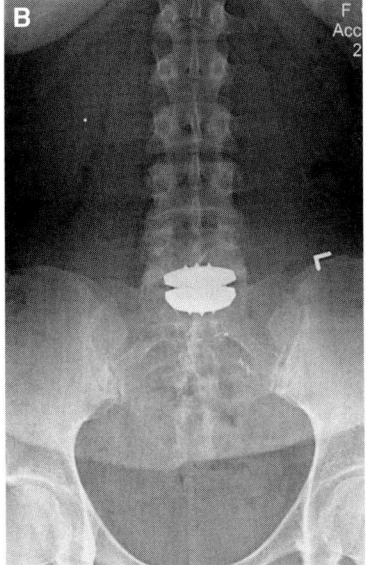

Fig. 4. (*A*, *B*) Lateral and anteroposterior view of Charite prosthesis placed in patient with L5-S1 disc disease.

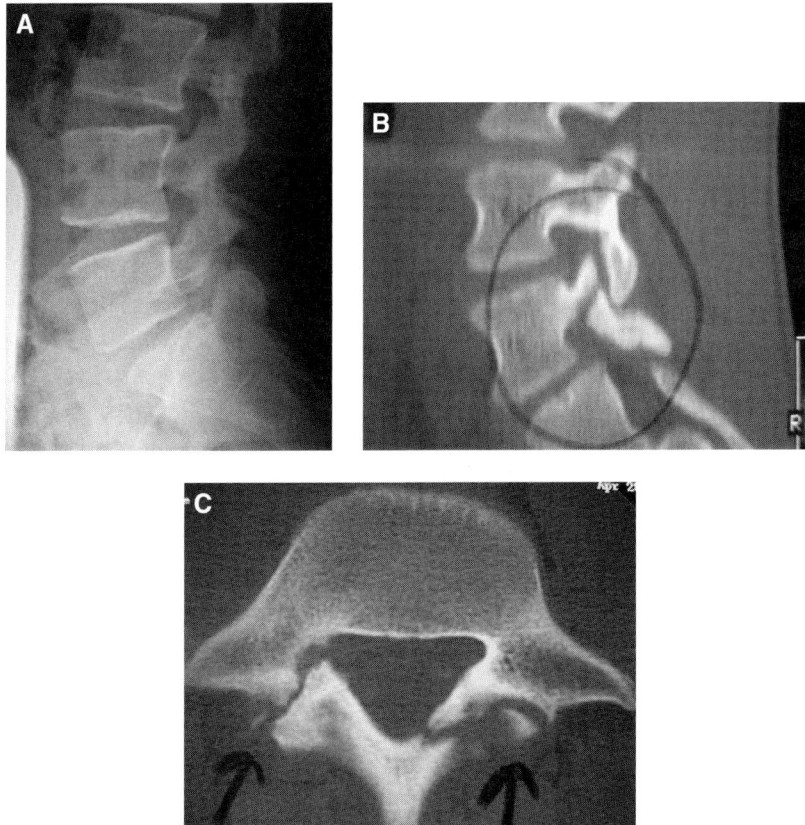

Fig. 5. (*A–C*) Pateint with spondylolysis who is not a candidate for artificial disc replacement.

our institution. This is one of the most critical parts of the operation with potentially disastrous complications (Please refer to complications section). Safe mobilization of the iliac vessels and adequate exposure of the intervertebral disc space can enhance the accuracy of the device placement as well as minimizing vascular complication during the implantation. Preoperative imaging with MRI and CT scan can help in identifying the vascular anatomy as it relates to the spinal segment receiving the artificial disc. Calcifications of the vessels are important to identify as well as any inflammatory process or protruding osteophytes at the disc level.

Radiographic measurements

Preoperative anteroposterior and lateral radiographs (including flexion and extension views) are obtained to evaluate segmental stability and motion as well as identifying transitional vertebrae, which may lead to incorrect localization intraoperatively. Radiographs need to be carefully examined to rule out occult spondylolysis. Oblique views or CT scans are obtained for further evaluation as needed. Posterior disc height at nondegenerated adjacent levels (generally one or two levels above the diseased level) must also be assessed to get an idea of normal disc height and the limit of maximum intraoperative distraction.

Operating room preparation

A radiolucent table that enables the use of an intraoperative C-arm image intensifier must be used. The lower lumbar spine should be adequately visualized in both AP and lateral views for safe and proper prosthetic placement. Furthermore, the operating table should allow flexion/extension of the lower spine intraoperatively. Lumbar extension may be needed (especially at L4/5 level) to perform adequate discectomy in a completely collapsed disc space as well during the anterior implant insertion. We use the Skytron 3100 operating table, which is equipped with a kidney rest that can be raised to increase lumbar lordosis when needed. We also prefer bringing the c-arm before prepping the patient to ensure adequate visualization of the disc space. The kidney rest is partially raised directly under the disc space to allow anterior opening of the disc, which will facilitate insertion of the prosthesis.

Operative technique

Positioning

The patient is placed supine on an operating table, and general endotracheal anesthesia is induced by the anesthesiologist. Prophylactic antibiotic is administered intravenously 30 minutes before the incision time. SSEP/ EMG as well as bilateral TEDs and SCDs are used in all cases. EMG abnormalities sometimes occur with left iliac vessel retraction in L4-5 cases secondary to ischemia. These potentials are also useful in assessing potential nerve irritation or injury from displaced osteophytes, which may occur during the endplate preparation or impaction phase of the procedure. Before the skin is prepared, the C-arm is brought in and the desired level is visualized on AP/lateral views and the planned incision is marked.

Surgical approach

After the abdomen is prepared and draped in the usual fashion, a transverse or vertical skin incision is made and a retroperitoneal dissection is performed to expose the desired level. The anterior rectus sheath is incised longitudinally and the rectus muscle on the left is retracted from the midline. The posterior rectus sheath and transversalis fascia are incised longitudinally. The transversalis fascia can be separated from the underlying peritoneal lining by finger dissection below the arcuate line, which is the inferior extent of the transversalis fascia. Using this technique, blunt dissection is used to dissect the peritoneum from left to right until the midline vascular structures and spine is identified by palpation. For exposure of an interspace above the aorta/vena cava bifurcation (eg, L4-L5), left-to-right dissection is performed and the vasculature is retracted to the right side after ligating segmental vessels. For the exposure of an interspace below the bifurcation (eg, L5-S1), left and right iliac vessels are retracted to their respective sides. Avoidance of monopolar cauterization and use of gentle dissection with sweeping of tissues away from the spine will minimize the chance of sympathetic plexus injury, which can lead to retrograde ejaculation in the male patient. For retraction, we prefer the use of the Omnitract, which uses renal blades of varying depths and anchors to the operating table for fixed retraction. Depending on the surgeon preference, alternative retraction techniques can be used, such as Wiley retractors for hand held retraction or anchorage of four instruments (such as sharp Homan's retractors) in the upper and lower vertebral bodies. It is important to obtain wide exposure and to visualize the width of the intervertebral space and up to the mid body of the level above and below the operating disc space. The iliac vessels must be retracted with the retractor blades out of the operating field. The left iliac vein has the tendency to creep under the blade and enter the field, which increases the risk of vascular injury. The surgeon must be cognizant of the location of the vessels and their safety throughout the case. Compared with anterior spinal fusion techniques, a greater side-to-side exposure is required for artificial disc replacement to allow for placement of larger size implants. Larger surface area coverage of the vertebral endplate is optimal for long-term success and in decreasing endplate subsidence.

Prosthetic implantation

Identification of the center of the vertebral body in coronal view

A spinal needle is placed in the middle of the disc and its location is verified under an AP view of an image intensifier. Adjustments are made and the radiolucent trial alignment guide is subsequently used to confirm midline position. This is followed by placement of 3.5-mm fully threaded cancellous screw-pin, 12 mm in length, in the cephalad vertebrae body, about 5 mm above the anterior lip. The screw is tapped gently with a mallet and then advanced (Figs. 6, 7).

Anterior annulotomy

A long handled 10-blade is used to perform the anterior annulotomy. An H-type incision is made by making the first cut in the center of the disc from rostral to caudal direction. Once the bony surface is reached, the blade is turned sideways and the superior/inferior annular attachments are incised bilaterally. The incision is taken laterally as far as the width of the anterior vertebral body, and an annular open book flap is created on both sides. A suture is placed at two ends of the flap and taken outside the wound secured with hemostats.

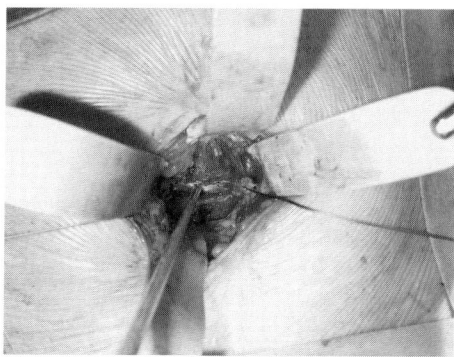

Fig. 6. Intraoperative view of trial sizer in place.

Complete discectomy

Cobb elevators, curettes, pituitary rongeurs, and kerrisons are used to perform a complete discectomy in a standard fashion. The kidney rest can be raised to open up the anterior disc space especially at the L4-5 level. Unlike spinal fusion surgery, disc material must be removed to the posterior annulus as well as removing any posterior osteophytes that may block the insertion of the prosthesis. The posterior aspect of the prosthesis will sit on the hard cortical bone of the posterior ring apophysis so it is imperative that posterior disc material be removed for easier insertion. Endplate preparation is also done using curettes to flatten any irregularities in the bony endplate. Osteotomy using osteotomes is not performed as it creates bleeding and can result in heterotopic bone formation as described by other investigators [6].

Parallel disc distraction

The central spreading distractor is placed in the disc space by using lateral fluoroscopy, and gentle distraction is applied. Posterior distraction should not exceed the normal posterior disc height of the levels above. In a severely collapsed disc space, the posterior longitudinal ligament as well as the posterior annulus may tear and a pop may be heard. Occasionally, posterior epidural venous bleeding is encountered for which hemostatic sponges are packed in the posterior disc space and left undisturbed for 3 to 5 minutes. Next, calibrated T-handle spreaders are introduced into the center of the endplate in a parallel fashion and then turned 90 degrees with the dominant hand as the contralateral hand places constant distraction force on the central distracting device. Distracting is started with size 7.5 mm and increased to 8.5 mm and then 9.5 mm, if a 9.5 mm polyethylene core is to be implanted.

Endplate templating. Different sized "lollipop" trials are used to determine implant size, and lateral fluoroscopy is used to ensure ~80% endplate coverage, the ability to place the implant in the ideal anatomic position (with the center of the implant being 0 to 3 mm posterior to the mid vertebral body), and stopping 2 to 3 mm short of the posterior vertebral border (Fig. 8).

Broaching

Broaching is performed with a grooved driver placed in the center of the body and driven posteriorly using a mallet. The anterior and posterior teeth of this instrument correspond to the teeth on the prosthesis. Lateral radiograph is taken to make certain that the instrument can be driven just short of the posterior edge of the inferior vertebral vertebral border. This generally ensures that the final implant will be inserted with appropriate predistraction of the interspace (Fig. 9).

Radiolucent trial guides. Radiolucent trial guides are used to establish the total angle of the combined superior and inferior endplates plus the core. For size 2 and 3 implants the guide assumes the addition of a 7.5 mm core and for size 4 and 5 prosthesis, the trial guide adds the 8.5mm height to approximate the footprint of the final prosthesis. Generally, there should not be a difference of more than 5 mm between the angled prosthesis placed at the superior endplate compared the inferior endplate device with the larger device placed at the inferior endplate. AP and lateral fluoroscopic images are taken with the

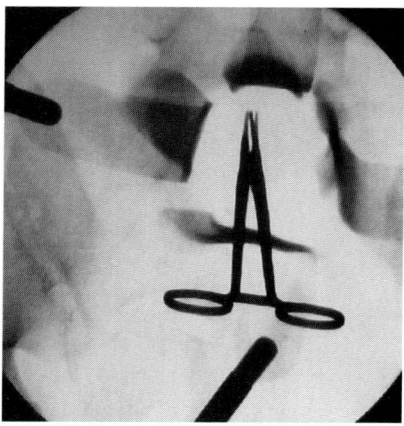

Fig. 7. Anteroposterior x-ray with marker in place to identify the midline.

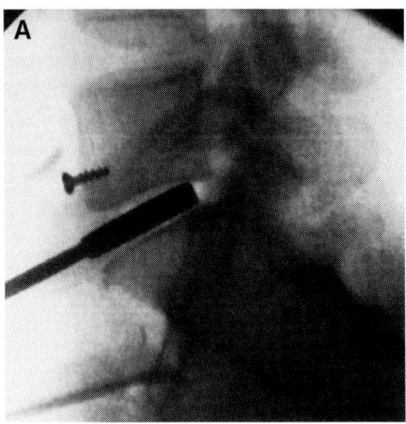 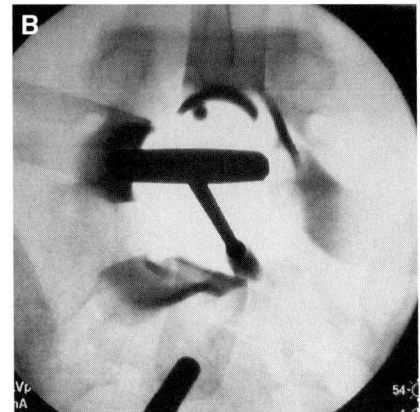

Fig. 8. (*A, B*) Lateral x-ray with "lollipop sizer" in place to assess proper implant size.

trial guide in place to assess the proper lordosis, as well as the centering in the AP projection and 2mm behind the midline in the lateral radiograph view. A screw is then placed in the midline so that the prosthesis can be inserted along this line (Fig. 10).

Prosthesis implantation. The prosthesis is correctly placed on the driver and implanted using a mallet under lateral C-arm fluoroscopy. It is important to align the implant parallel to the endplate during placement. Any deviation from parallelism can cause violation of the upper or the lower endplate, which can lead to improper implant placement and subsequent subsidence. Once the posterior tip of the prosthesis passes the middle of the vertebral body, the kidney rest is lowered to allow the disc space to return to its natural position. Ideally, the center of the prosthesis should be about 0 to 3 mm posterior to the midline of the vertebral body. This position most accurately simulates the anatomic instantaneous axis

of rotation. As the implant is driven posteriorly, the posterior teeth will hit the posterior apophyseal ring, or the posterior lip of the vertebral body, and it will come to a stop. Aggressive impaction should be avoided at this point as it may cause fracture of the posterior apophyseal ring. If there is difficulty inserting the implant, the implant should be removed and the broach reinserted and tapped to the posterior edge of the inferior vertebral body to ensure appropriate distraction (Fig. 11).

Sliding core insertion. The implant is distracted enough to insert the polyethylene core in the center of the implant followed by release of the distraction. Penfield four is used to ensure the core rotates freely followed by removal of the driver (Fig. 12).

Final implant positioning. The lateral radiograph should show the implant with the center 1 to 3 mm posterior to the middle of the vertebra and short of the posterior edge of the vertebral body about 3 mm. An AP view is then obtained before to check midline alignment. The prosthesis needs to be within 0 to 3 mm of the lateral borders of the spinous process. If the implant is off midline by more than 3 mm, the implant should be removed and repositioned unless technical difficulties are encountered. Next, the upper and lower teeth are driven further into the endplate using an impactor (Figs. 13, 14).

Annular closure. Although it has not shown to have any biomechanical advantage, anterior annular closure can be performed using a number one absorbable suture. The center marking screw is taken out using a screwdriver, and the void is filled with small amount of bone wax to obtain hemostasis. Wound is

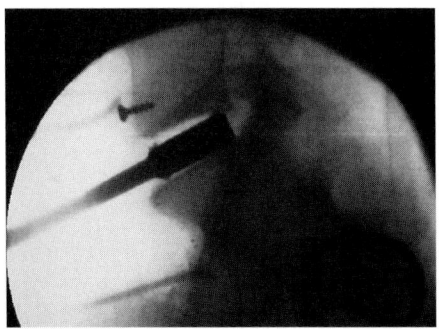

Fig. 9. Broach is inserted to create grooves and assess predistraction prior to implant insertion.

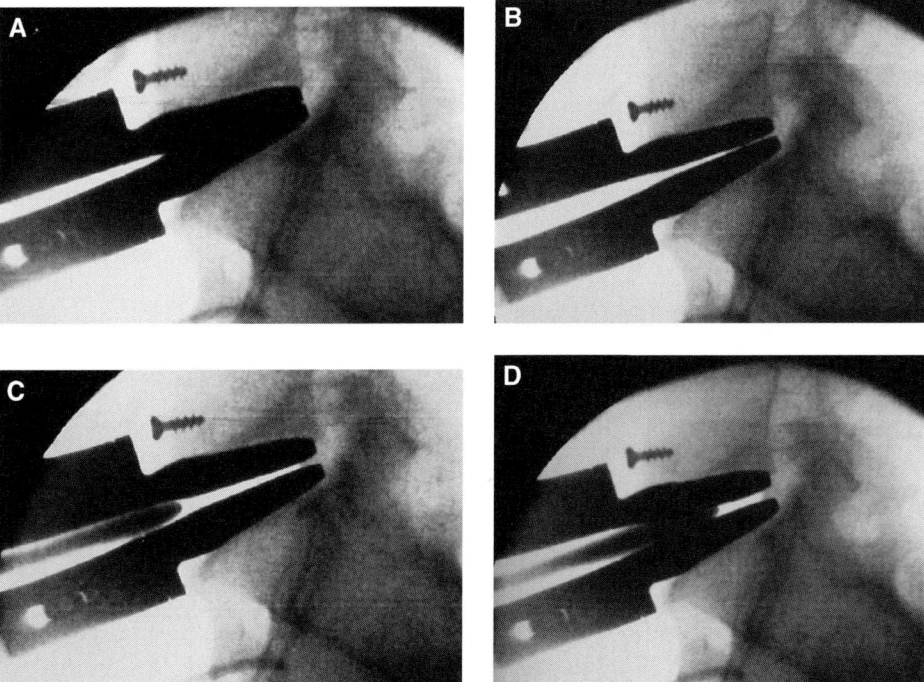

Fig. 10. (A–D) Lordotic trials are used to assess the proper implant size and angle to be used.

copiously irrigated followed by closure of the rectus fascia, subcutaneous fascia, and the skin using absorbable sutures (Fig. 15).

Immediate postoperative period

Pain management

Ketorolac (Toradol) 30 mg IV is given every 8 hours for total of three doses with the first dose given at the end of the case. Alternatively, a Cox-2 inhibitor can be given with a sip of water in the preoperative holding area before surgery. This has the advantage of avoiding platelet aggregation effects and decreasing GI side effects compared with Toradol. Oral opioid analgesic combinations are used on p.r.n. bases with intravenous opioid agonist, such as morphine sulfate or hydromorphone, for breakthrough pain only. We avoid using pain controlled administration (PCA) as it delays postoperative bowel recovery and rehabilitation. Patients are discharged on oral opioid analgesic combinations on p.r.n basis as well as daily oral nonsteroidal anti-inflammatory medication for 4 weeks.

Diet

With presence of bowel sounds, sips of liquid are started 6 hours after surgery and advanced to liquid diet on the first postoperative day as tolerated. Patients can be discharged home on postoperative day 1 on liquid diet with clear instructions on how to advance diet at home.

Activity

Patients are allowed to sit up, get out of bed, and walk with assistance.

Rehabilitation

The postoperative rehabilitation program for patients with the Charité Artificial Disc is as follows:

- *<3 weeks:* Lumbar flexion and cardiovascular exercises are permitted during this immediate postoperative period with restriction on rotation and lumbar extension.
- *3–6 weeks:* Lumbar rotation can be started.

- *6–12 weeks:* Lumbar extension can be performed at this point unless the initial implant placement is in >10 degrees of divergent for which extension should be restricted for 12 weeks. With time, there is increased scar formation over the anterior annulus, which provides a blockage to anterior implant dislocation. Anterior abdominal exercises as well as truncal stabilization can begin during this period.
- *>12 weeks:* Return to sports must be individualized and determined by the treating surgeon. Contact sports and high impact activities that would place a large stress on the endplates should be avoided.

Results

In 1997, Lemaire et al [11] reported on their clinical experience with the lumbar Charité Artificial Disc in France. A total of 105 cases, with a mean follow-up of 51 months, was reviewed, which showed 79% of the patients with excellent results and 87% returned to work. Factors leading to failure were listed as posterior facet arthritis, osteoporosis, structural deformities, and secondary facet pain.

The US prospective randomized FDA trial on the Charité Artificial Disc IDE study for one-level lumbar disc disease with a minimum of 2-year follow-up was completed in December 2003. A total of 375 patients was enrolled in 15 investigational US sites with a 2:1 randomization of Charité:BAK after completion of 71 training cases (five training case/site). One third of patients were randomized with the BAK anterior interbody fusion device (n = 99) and two thirds of patients with the Charité Artificial Disc (n = 205). Postoperative follow-up was performed at 3 months, 6 months, 12 months, and 24 months. Data were collected on 276 patients (71 training cases and 205 randomized) who received the artificial disc and 99 BAK cases. Minimum follow-up period was 2 years with 91% of patients returning at 2 years. Mean surgery time was significantly improved in the randomized group (110.8 minutes) compared with the initial training group (141.9 minutes), $P < 0.001$. Mean operative time and blood loss was similar for both the BAK and Artificial Disc group. The length of stay was less in the artificial disc group (3.7 versus 4.3 days). VAS pain scores and ODI improved significantly in both groups with the Charite group experiencing a significantly greater improvement at 6 week, 3 months, 6 months, and 1 year. Patient satisfaction was 93% with the Charite prosthesis compared with 81% satisfaction for the BAK spinal fusion procedure at 1 year following the procedure. At the end of 24 months, 13% of BAK fusions were very dissatisfied with the procedure compared with only 2% of the disc replacement patients. Asked if they would choose the same treatment, at 24 months following the procedure, 82% of the Charite artificial disc group said yes and only 65% of the fusion cases would have the procedure repeated. There was a higher rate of complications in the training group compared with the randomized group and a lower complication rate in the groups with greater than 10 cases. Operative time was also less in the high enrolling sites (3.5 days for high enrolling sites compared with 4.5 days for the low enrolling sites). Major complications (vessel injury, implant displacement, or neurologic injury) were less than 1% in both BAK and Charite groups.

We evaluated our single-site experience with the Charité Artificial Disc on 100 consecutive patients with minimum of 6 months follow-up (range: 6 to 24 months). The first 13 patients were part of the 2:1 Charité: BAK FDA randomized trial and the following 88 patients were part of the continued access nonrandomized Investigational Drug Exemption (IDE) group. There were 54 males and 46 females with the prosthesis placed at L4-5 in 32 patients and at L5-S1 in 68 patients. VAS and ODI scores were recorded for all patients preoperatively and postoperatively at 6 weeks, 3, 6, 12, and 24 months. The mean preoperative VAS of 73.2 (S.D. 14.5) was improved to 39.2 (S.D. 26.4) at 6 weeks postoperatively ($P < 0.001$, paired t-test) and was maintained at 3, 6 months, and for those patients reaching 12 months ($P < 0.001$) and 24 months ($P < 0.001$) of follow-up. The mean preoperative ODI score was 53.4 (S.D. 13.4) and improved to 37.6 (S.D. 18.6, $P < 0.001$, paired t-test) at 6 weeks and sustained at 3, 6, 12, and 24 months follow-up visits. There was no statistical difference in outcome when L4-L5 was compared with L5-S1. Seven patients in this series experienced complications related to the implant. Three patients had their implants removed after anterior migration of the prosthesis in the early postoperative time period. One of the prosthetic dislocations occurred in a patient who was noncompliant with postoperative rehabilitation protocol and performed hyperextension exercise 1 week after surgery.

Fig. 11. (*A–F*) Implant is loaded on trays and inserted into the pre-distracted disc space. Controlled distraction is performed to permit insertion of core. (*A–C, E, F: Courtesy of* DePuy Spine, Raynham, MA; with permission.)

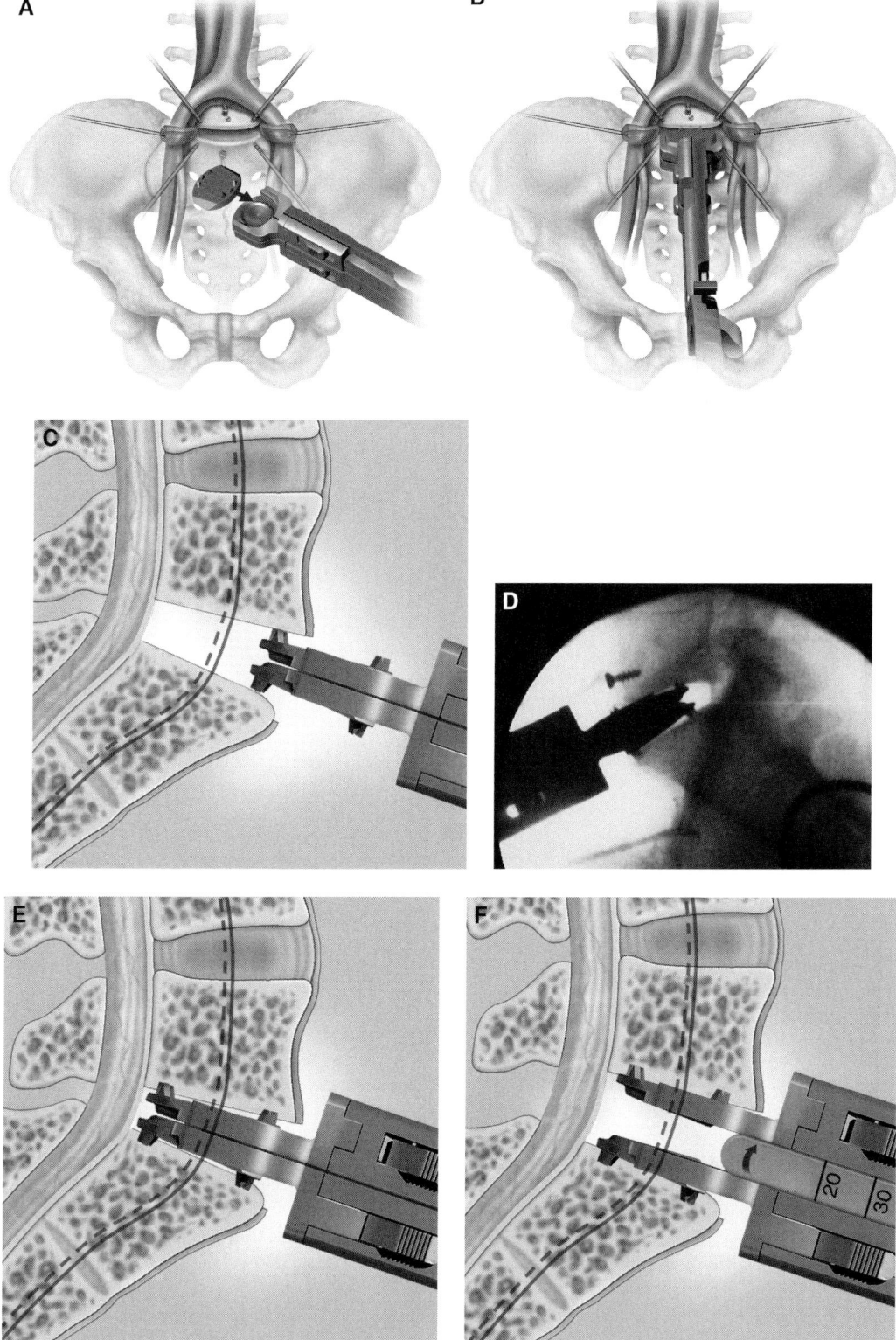

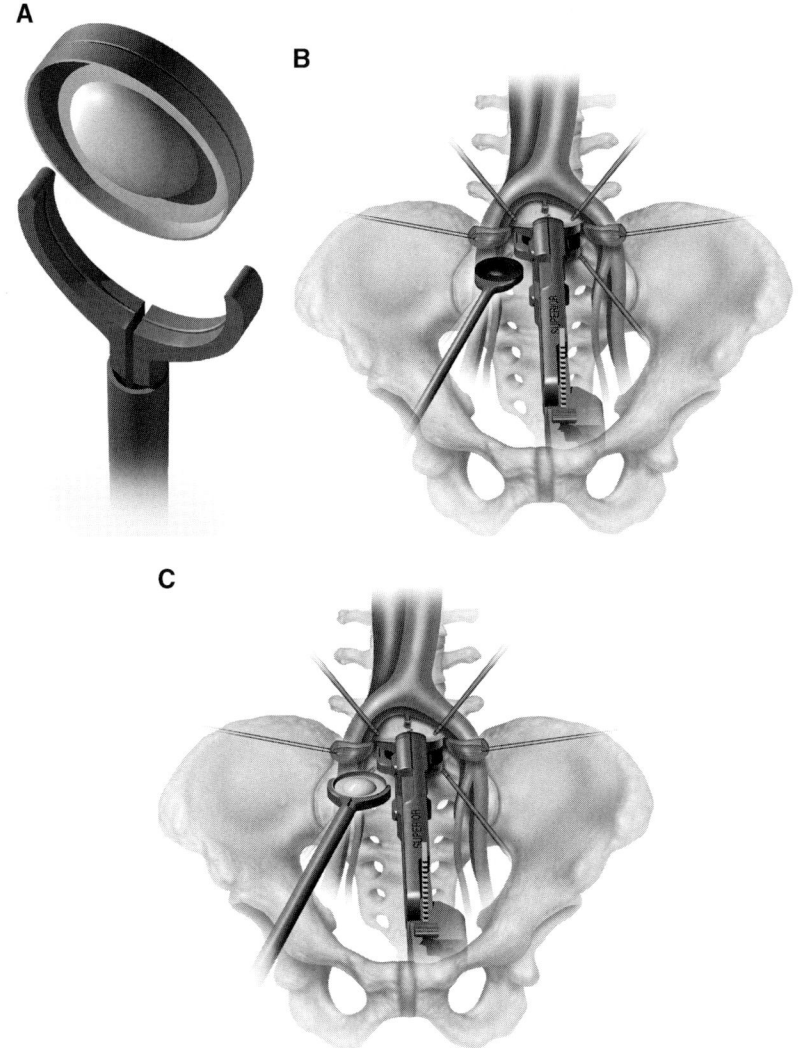

Fig. 12. (*A*–*C*) Core is loaded on holer and inserted into disc space after proper sizing. Minimum sizes are 7.5 mm for size 3 implants and 8.5 mm for implant size 4 and 5. (*Courtesy of* DePuy Spine, Raynham, MA; with permission.)

An anterior displacement occurred in one patient with no inciting event on postoperative day 12. This complication was attributed to the steep sacral inclination and slight anterior position of the implant. Two of the patients underwent a repeat anterior retroperitoneal approach and removal of the prosthesis followed by anterior interbody fusion and posterior spinal fusion with instrumentation. The third patient had an exchange prosthesis of a smaller size and continues to do well 1 year later. Two patients experienced endplate fractures with resulting radicular pain requiring posterior foraminotomy. Two additional patients who had previously undergone laminotomy fractured the facet joint on the side of the previous laminotomy at 3 weeks and 9 months respectively. Two additional patients underwent posterior spinal fusion and instrumentation due to continued low back pain with the device in situ at 6 months and 20 months postoperatively.

Complications

Surgical approach–related complications

The most important factor in minimizing complications is to have an experienced vascular or a general surgeon, who is familiar with anterior lumbar

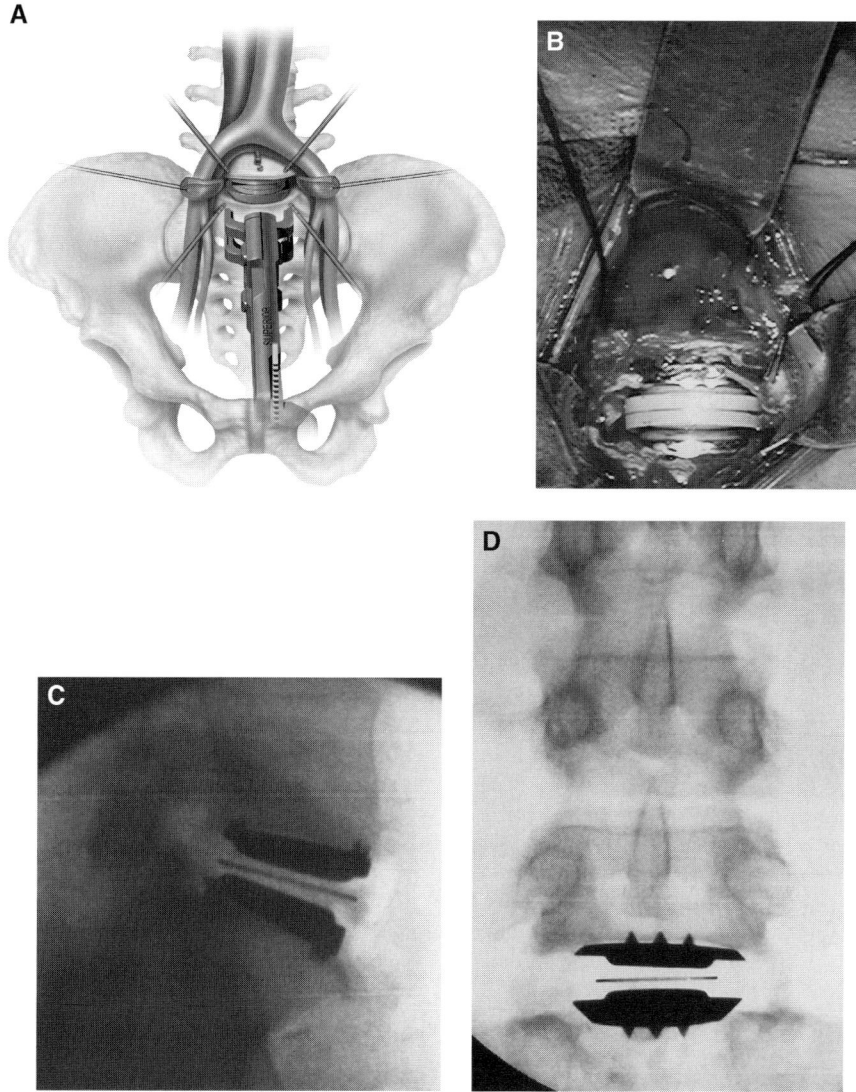

Fig. 13. (*A–D*) Final positioning of implant at L5-S1 showing horizontalization of the endplate at S1 using a 10-degree implant. (*A: Courtesy of* DePuy Spine, Raynham, MA; with permission.)

exposures, perform the surgical approach. However, minor as well as major complications can still occur during both the surgical approach and the implantation. Therefore, extreme diligence and attention to detail throughout the entire procedure cannot be overemphasized. Although both transperitoneal and retroperitoneal approaches may be used, most surgeons prefer the latter approach due to its lower morbidity. With the transperitoneal approach, there is higher risk of postoperative ileus, small bowel obstruction, and retrograde ejaculations.

With the retroperitoneal approach, inadvertent peritoneal tissue penetration may occur which can be safely sutured closed. Postoperative ileus can still occur even without peritoneal tissue violation. It has been our experience that the use of PCA dramatically slows down the bowel recovery and therefore we have abandoned its use for these procedures.

Vena cava or left iliac vein injury can occur during surgical dissection as well as implantation. Although this is not a common complication when an experienced access surgeon performs the approach, these injuries can cause sever morbidity and even mortality. Therefore, protection of the vessels with blunt retractors after dissection is very important. The surgeon must be cognizant of the location and the safety of the

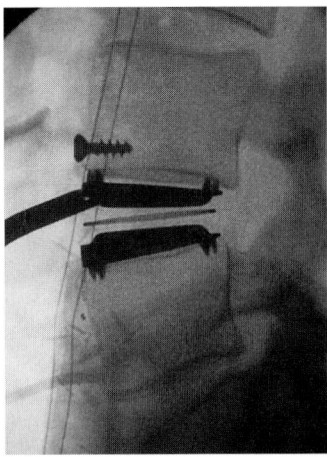

Fig. 14. Spikes are tapped into the endplate to further recess the implant.

vessels through out the entire procedure. Left iliac deep vein venous thrombosis and pelvic phlebitis can occur from prolonged retraction. Although this is a rare complication some surgeons place a pulse oximeter on the left toe to monitor the blood flow.

With the anterior lumbar approach, male patients have a small risk of postoperative retrograde ejaculation that is often transient but may be permanent. Due to the close proximity of the sympathetic plexus, manipulation or retraction of the chain may also cause the sympathetic effect. This could cause sensation of a warmer left leg compared with the contralateral side. With retroperitoneal approach, careful dissection, and judicious use of monopolar electrocautery, the risk of these complications is minimized. At our institution, we have not experienced this complication in the 70 patients who have undergone the lumbar total disc replacement.

Left ureter injury can occur during retroperitoneal approach with a higher risk during revision surgery. Urethral stent may be beneficial in presence of scar tissue and can be performed by a urologist.

Adhering to strict sterile technique and maintenance of hemostasis, respectively, can minimize the risk of infection and deep hematoma. Careful closure of the rectus fascia can prevent abdominal hernias.

Immediate complications of implantation

During central distraction and restoration of the disc height and lordosis, the following complications may be encountered. Epidural venous bleeding can occur, especially with distraction of a collapsed disc space, which can be controlled by packing hemostatic sponges in the posterior disc space and left undisturbed for 3 to 5 minutes.

Postoperative radicular pain can result from stretching the exiting nerve root during distraction of a previously posterior lumbar surgery with perineuronal scarring or overdistraction. This is often transient and resolved with conservative management. Overdistraction can be avoided by restoring the posterior disc height to its normal level as judged by the adjacent segments with a normal disc height. Although restoration of the disc height can offload the impacted posterior facets when maintained after placement of the prosthesis, intraoperative overdistraction with central spreader can also theoretically disrupt the posterior facet capsule and act as a source of pain postoperatively (Fig. 16).

Malpositioning of the implant in the coronal as well as sagittal plane should be avoided as it may affect the patient outcome. The ideal lateral placement is the center of the prosthesis 0 to 3 mm posterior to the center of the vertebral body in the sagittal plane. This position closely simulates the anatomic IAR. In the coronal plane, the implant should also be placed in the center of the vertebral body Radiographically, the middle tooth of the implant in the AP view should be within 0 to 3 mm of the spinous process. In our reviewed series of 40 patients with minimum of 6-month follow-up, there was a negative correlation between ideal AP positioning and patient satisfaction if the AP alignment was outside the 3 mm range.

It is important to remember that the vertebral body consists of dense cortical apophyseal ring at the

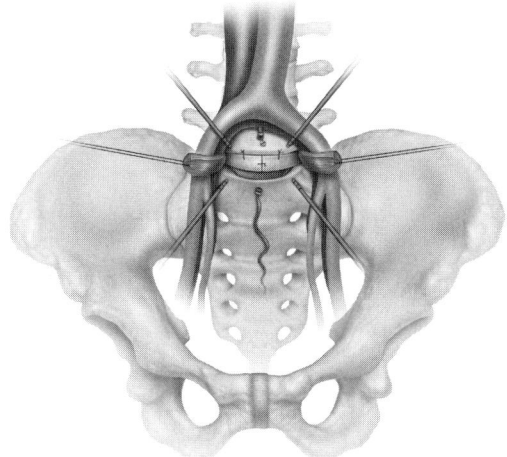

Fig. 15. Anterior longitudinal ligament can be sutured in place but is not necessary. (*Courtesy of* DePuy Spine, Raynham, MA; with permission.)

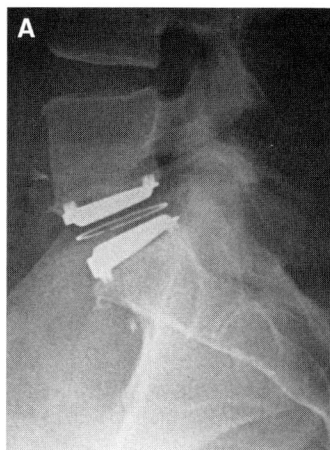 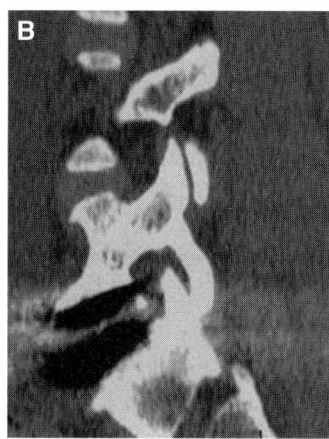

Fig. 16. (*A, B*) Implant at L5-S1 showing more distraction than necessary and open facet from over-lordosing the patient. Patient complained of back and buttock pain that resolved in 8 weeks.

periphery and cartilaginous endplate in the center. Therefore, the posterior apophyseal ring acts as a safety stop preventing the prosthesis from entering the canal during implantation. As the implant is impacted in the disc space under lateral fluoroscopy, the posterior teeth of the prosthesis will come in contact with the dense cortical posterior apophyseal ring and high level of resistance is felt. If a large implant is chosen with >90% lateral endplate coverage, it becomes harder to drive the prosthesis in the ideal position and aggressive attempts at driving the prosthesis further posterior can cause fracture of the posterior apophyseal ring into the canal. Therefore it is important to choose the right size implant during templating that provides the largest endplate coverage and that it can also be placed in the ideal anatomic position, keeping in mind that the implant has to stop 2 to 3 mm short of the posterior vertebral border (Fig. 17).

Anterior implant subluxation or dislocation is often the result of poor implant placement (anterior to the mid-sagittal line of the vertebral body) and patient's noncompliance with postoperative activity restrictions such as hyperextension, or large lumbosacral angle. Placing the implant with >15° of divergence or segmental lordosis increased the risk of dislocation and should be avoided. This position allows minimal implant extension, which can lead to a dislocation if a patient continues lumbar extension beyond this limit. This can be avoided by placing oblique or augmented endplates to obtain parallel endplates. Vertical endplate is also a risk factor for implant dislocation, which can due to a large lumbosacral angle or poor implant placement by violating the endplate during placement. Currently, we routinely use inferior endplate augmentation at L5-S1 to decrease the anterior disc height and obtain parallelism. Anterior dislocation in the immediate postoperative period can be taken back to surgery for revision easier than with late dislocation due to lack of well-formed scar tissue (Fig. 18).

Long-term complications of implantation

Subsidence of the prosthesis into the vertebral body can occur as a result of asymmetric implantation, under sizing of the implant and intraoperative endplate violation. This complication may cause persistent activity-related back pain and may require a posterior spinal fusion. With use of lateral fluoroscopy during implantation, endplate violation can be avoided by ensuring that the prosthesis is getting inserted parallel to the endplates. This is sometimes hard to accomplish at L5-S1 with presence of large lumbosacral angle where the surgeon's hand needs to be lowered caudally significantly. The inferior retractors may also abut against the hand and their positions may need to be adjusted (Fig. 19).

Although some investigators have reported partial or total heterotopic ossification surrounding the prosthesis rendering in immobile [12], 6% incidence has been reported at 2 years (with no bridging of osteophytes) in the US prospective randomized trial. Even though cause of heterotopic ossification is multifactorial, osseous bleeding from osteotomies may be a contributing factor to heterotopic ossification formation. We do not perform endplate osteotomies, as some surgeons do, to obtain greater

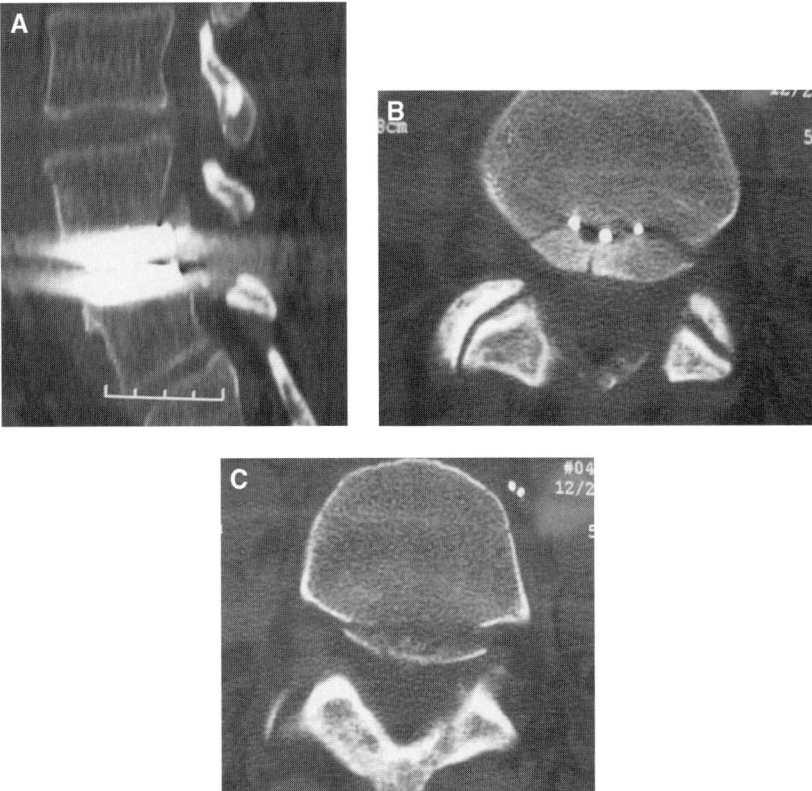

Fig. 17. (*A–C*) Endplate fracture associated with implant impaction related to insufficient predistraction. The patient complained of postoperative radiculopathy requiring posterior foraminotomy and partial removal of bone fragment.

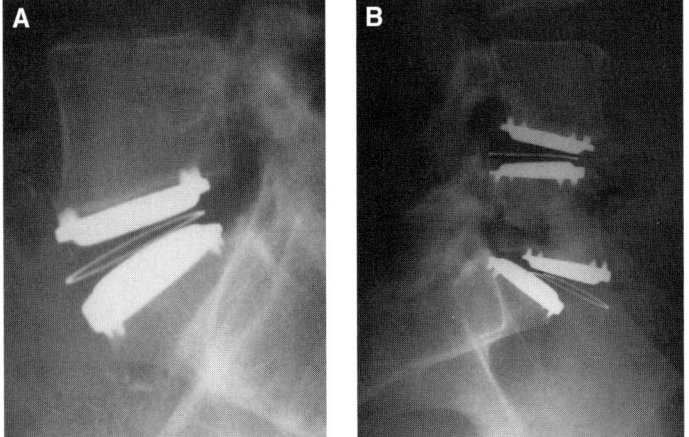

Fig. 18. (*A*) Anterior position of implant at L5-S1, which can lead to (*B*) anterior dislocation, which occurred in this two level case 3 weeks after surgery requiring implant removal and fusion at L5-S1.

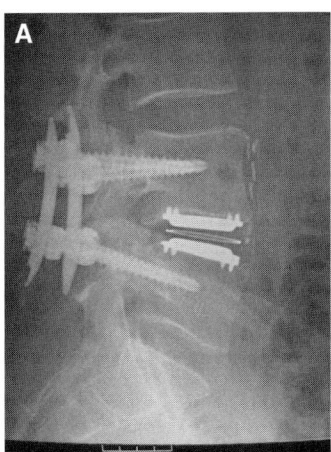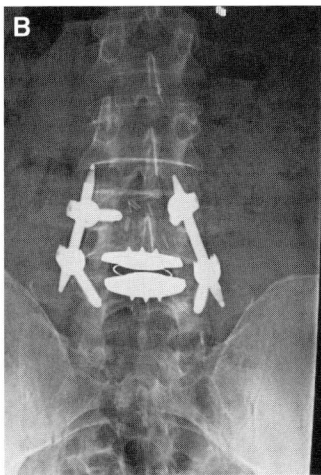

Fig. 19. (A, B) Posterior fusion and instrumentation is done for a patient who developed acute back pain following a hyperextension exercise leading to endplate fracture and chronic pain.

area of contact between the implant and the endplate. Cox-2 nonsteroidal anti-inflammatory medication is routinely prescribed in the postoperative time period to decrease pain and minimize heterotopic bone formation.

Infection of the implant, which has not been reported in the randomized Charite study in the United States, can be very difficult to treat and its management would be similar to any other intervertebral body fusion device. Clearly, as with management of a late implant dislocation, anterior approach to the disc space is most challenging aspect of the re-operations. In Europe, the anterolateral approach is used at L4-5 and an osteoligamentous flap is raised under the iliac vessels to avoid difficult dissection of the vessels from the anterior disc space.

Persistent low back pain can be secondary to poor patient selection, inaccurate diagnosis, and poor implant placement. Posterior spinal fusion with instrumentation can be performed as a salvage opera-

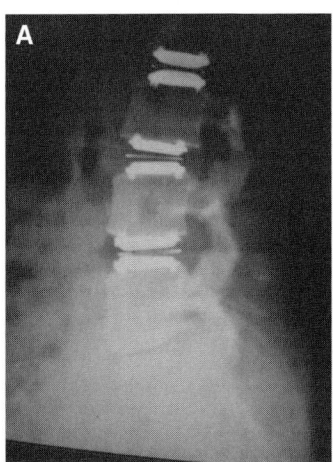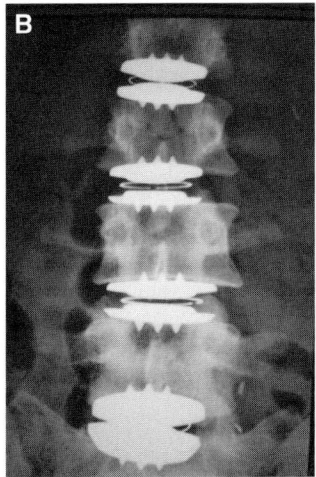

Fig. 20. (A, B) Multilevel artificial disc case performed in South America.

tion for those patients with posterior facet pathology or persistent pain of unknown cause.

Summary

In the past, low back pain secondary to degenerative disc disease was treated nonoperatively as surgical treatment often led to unsatisfactory results. With advances in technology in the past 2 decades, spinal arthrodesis is used by many spine surgeons for patients in whom nonoperative management has failed. However, several investigators have raised concern regarding long-term effect of lumbar fusion (>10 to 15 years) as it may place more stress on the adjacent levels causing early degeneration [6,7,11,13]. Moreover, the attractive idea of preserving lumbar motion and at the same time treating discogenic back pain has sparked a great enthusiasm among many investigators to design disc implants that most closely simulate the normal biomechanics of the lumbar disc [5,10].

The Charité Artificial Disc preserves segmental motion as well as the instant axis of rotation of the lumbar spine. The unconstrained three-component feature of the implant allows restoration of the functional sagittal lordosis and balance. To date, many European studies as well as early US clinical results have showed >70% satisfactory results with the use of this device [1–7]. The most important factors in obtaining good results are proper surgical indication, as the single most critical factor, followed by accurate implant placement (Fig. 20).

Although the early clinical results of lumbar total disc replacements are promising, long-term results with adequate follow-up are needed to adequately assess the efficacy of lumbar disc replacement in selected patients with discogenic low back pain. Additionally, long-term issues such as polyethylene wear and its behavior on the surrounding structures, longevity of the implant, the effect of motion sparing device on the adjacent as well as on the same segment, and the results of revision surgeries for failed implants will be better defined in the future [14–16]. Before embarking on the use of the prosthesis, the reader is advised to stay up to date with the literature on lumbar total disc replacement outcome studies, as with use of any other new investigational device, to offer patients the most sensible treatment option at any time period.

References

[1] Büttner-Janz K, Hochshuler SH, McAfee PC. The artificial disc. Hamburg, Germany: Waldemar Link GmbH & Co.; 2003.

[2] Cinotti G, David T, Postacchini F. Results of disc prosthesis after a minimum follow-up period of 2 years. Spine 1996;21(8):995–1000.

[3] Hochschuler SH, Ohnmeiss DD, Guyer RD, Blumenthal SL. Artificial disc: preliminary results of a prospective study in the United States. Eur Spine J 2002; 11(Suppl 2):S106–10.

[4] Kim WJ, Lee SH, Kim SS, Lee C. Treatment of juxtafusional degeneration with artificial disc replacement (ADR): preliminary results of an ongoing prospective study. JSDT 2003;16(4):390–7.

[5] Link HD. History, design, and biomechanics of the Link SB Charité artificial disc. Eur Spine J 2002; 11;S98–105.

[6] McAfee PC, Fedder IL, Saiedy S, et al. SB Charité disc replacement: report of 60 prospective randomized cases in US center. JSDT 2003;16(4):424–43.

[7] Zeegers WS, Bohnen LMLJ, Laaper M, et al. Artificial disc replacement with the modular type SB Charité III: 2-year results in 50 prospectively studied patients. Eur Spine J 1999;8:210–7.

[8] Dooris AP, Goel VK, Grosland NM, et al. Load-sharing between anterior and posterior elements in lumbar motion segment implanted with an artificial disc. Spine 2001;26(6):E122–9.

[9] White AA, Panjabi MM. Clinical biomechanics of the spine. Philadelphia: Lippincott; 1990.

[10] Bao QB, McCullen GM, Higham PA, et al. The artificial disc: theory, design and materials. Biomaterials 1996;17(12):1157–67.

[11] Lemaire JP, Skalli W, Lavaste F, et al. ntervertebral disc prosthesis. Results and prospects for the year 2000. CORR 1997;337:64–76.

[12] McAfee PC, Cunningham BW, Devine J, et al. Classification of heterotopic ossification (HO) in artificial disk replacement. JSDT 2003;16(4):384–9.

[13] Lee CK. Accelerated degeneration of the segment adjacent to lumbar fusion. Spine 1988;13:375–7.

[14] Boden SD, Balderson RA, Heller JG, et al. Disc replacements: this time will we really cure low-back and neck pain? JBJS 2004;86-A:411–22.

[15] Van Ooij A, Oner FC, Verbout AJ. Complications of artificial disc replacement: a report of 27 patients with the SB Charite disc. JSDT 2003;6(4):369–83.

[16] Szpalski M, Gunzburg R, Mayer M. Spine arthroplasty: a historical review. Eur Spine J 2002;11(Suppl 2): S65–84.

Lumbar Partial Disc Replacement

Rudolf Bertagnoli, MD[a,*], Armin Karg, MSc[b], Sandra Voigt, MSc[b]

[a]*Spine Center, St.-Elisabeth-Klinikum, St.-Elisabeth-Str. 23, 94315 Straubing, Germany*
[b]*Spine Center Straubing, Obere Bachstrasse 30 a, 94315 Straubing, Germany*

Back pain is universally shared and causes many doctor visits around the world. About 40% of people aged 25 to 74 suffer from back pain. The consequences of impaired musculoskeletal conditions are drastic and expensive for the patients as well as for the economy: long duration of employee absenteeism, hospitalization, and disability. The number of patients is still increasing, and with it the need for better and optimal treatment options. Even though not all of the patients who suffer from natural disc degeneration need medical treatment, some patients require medical as well as clinical treatment to reduce their severe back pain.

Disc mechanics and physiology

The intervertebral disc has two important main functions: to provide cushioning and to allow the axial skeleton to remain flexible. Each intervertebral disc consists of two components: the multilayered fibers of the annulus fibrosus and the soft and gelatinous nucleus pulposus in the center.

The annulus consists of multiple laminations or plies [1]. The inelastic collagen fibers of every lamination attach to each adjacent vertebral body in a diagonal orientation [2]. The cushioning effect is created by the fibers and their laminations, which permit bulging under load.

Within the outer annulus, the content of fibers is around 90%; toward the center of the disc, the gel component increases; and in the center of the disc, the gel component is about 90% and the fibers only about 10%. The internal fibers of the annulus are not connected to the vertebrae but they provide substance to the nucleus mass.

The nucleus consists of collagens and proteoglycans. The proteoglycans provide the tissue with its stiffness and resistance against compression by their interactions with water [3,4]. The water-binding capacity of the nucleus depends on the presence of these hydrophilic proteins. Furthermore the water content varies depending on the external disc load. Under high load conditions, the water squeezes into the adjacent vertebral endplates and it returns under low load. This pumping mechanism is necessary to provide the metabolism to the vessel-free nucleus [5]. Consequently the water content is higher in the morning, after a rest, but in the evening the nucleus has lost some water and the thickness is not so high anymore. Also the composition of the nucleus changes as a result of the normal aging process: In youth the water content is about 80%, but due to a gradual change in the type of proteoglycans the nucleus is more fibrous by the third decade of life. Within this natural progress, the nucleus is usually significantly dehydrated and has lost its mucoid consistence by the fifth decade which explains the loss of height of older people.

Capillaries and free nerve endings, the pain transmitters, can be found only in the outer layers of the annulus. The nucleus and inner annulus are anaerobic, the nutritional exchange of intradiscal metabolites passes through the intact cartilaginous endplate and its channels. The process depends on osmotic differentials and diurnal pumping action. Under low load conditions at night fluid and nutrients are pulled

* Corresponding author.
  E-mail address: bertagnoli@pro-spine.com
  (R. Bertagnoli).

into the disc by the hydrophilic nucleus gel and under high load conditions during the day the byproducts exit through the endplate and into the capillary bed.

Under load, the semisolid nucleus pushes radially out from the center of the disc and causes the annulus to bulge [7,8]. By tensioning of the collagen fibers, the annulus dissipates the compressive forces. This lets the intervertebral disc operate as a cushion between each single vertebral body. During this process the inner as well as the outer margins of the annulus bulge outward. However, when the nucleus no longer functions properly, under similar loading the inner annulus bulges or folds inward as the outer margin bulges outward [9]. In case of desiccation of the layers between the laminations, the folding of the annulus can cause tears, delamination, and consequently weaken the disc. The appearance of tears may result in problems with internal disc metabolites. They can escape and reach the outer belt of the pain-transmitting free nerve endings or even the vertebral canal. Already very little quantities of anaerobic metabolites can lead to acute or chronic back or leg pain and little motion of the segment will cause severe pain to the patient. The exchange of wastes and nutrients as well as an intact annulus and nucleus are essential for a healthy and proper functioned disc.

Treating degenerative disc disease with a prosthetic nucleus

After failed conservative therapy, only discectomy and fusion exist as further treatment steps [10]. Discectomy is a good option for people with direct nerve root compression, inflammation, or vascular changes affecting the ganglion or root. But due to the mechanical component that also induces back pain, it is no solution for this component of discogenic low back pain. The segment gets less stable and less functional as more of the nucleus pulposus is removed [11].

Patients with degenerative back pain with failed conservative treatment have received further insufficient treatment, pain treatment, or as a surgical option, fusion surgery. Although fusion procedures relieve pain relatively well, they are very invasive treatments with a relatively high potential of complications, severe collateral damage of surrounding soft tissue structures, and create significant changes to the biomechanics of the segment by eliminating the segment function and mobility permanently. The literature supports a relatively high incidence of adjacent segment degeneration due to these biomechanical changes.

The nucleus pulposus seems to be the starting point of the degenerative cascade in many cases and should be a major treatment target [6]. The idea of partial disc replacement is to replace only the nucleus as the origin for the pain while restoring the biomechanical function of the disc and therefore also the function of the whole segment. Lumbar partial disc replacement is one opportunity to fill the therapy gap in the earlier stages of disc degeneration that exist between discectomy and fusion [12].

Development of nucleus replacement devices

In the early stages (late 1950s and early 1960s) of partial disc replacement, the nucleus pulposus space was instilled or replaced with polymethylmethacrylate (PMMA), silicon, or stainless steel ball bearings [13–15]. Due to a lack of knowledge about disc mechanics, such as pressure, range of motion, migration and subsidence issues, the results from these early procedures were not sufficiently acceptable and none of the devices obtained acceptance at that time.

The Fernstrom ball attempted to preserve motion by replacing the nucleus with stainless steel ball bearings and retaining most of the annulus fibrosis [15]. In general, the results for the Fernstrom ball were good for patients with sciatic pain. Less optimal results were noted for patients who suffered from spondylolisthesis and severe facet arthropathy. In most of the cases major subsidence occurred, causing bad clinical outcome.

About the same time, Nachemson [15] injected silicon and Hamby and Glaser [14] tried injecting PMMA into the disc but had flow control problems and poor outcome. The results of this early research provided a basis for the further development of a nucleus replacement, which would restore biomechanics and biology and prevent further degeneration of the disc.

In the early 1980s, available materials could tolerate the compression and shear forces expected in the disc space, but several devices failed at fatigue testing.

In the last few years, the understanding of the biomechanics of the disc and the degenerative cascade has been elucidated and that led to attempts to reproduce the biphasic and viscoelastic mechanical properties of the nucleus pulposus, using synthetic hydrogels. The hydrophilic nature of these polymers mimics the transport and biomechanical properties of the natural soft tissue, including the intervertebral disc [16,17]. For more than 15 years hydrogel-based

Table 1
Classification of nucleus disc replacement devices

Device	Material	Constrained and/or predefined geometry	Unconstrained devices	Injectable devices
Soft devices				
PDN	Hypan	x	–	–
PDN-SOLO				
NeuDisc	Hydrogel	x	–	–
DASCOR	Polyurethane	x	–	x
Newcleus	Polycarbonate urethane	–	x	–
Aquarelle	Polyvinyl alcohol	–	x	–
SINUX	Silicone	–	–	x
BioDisc	Protein hydrogel	–	–	x
NuCore	Silk elastin protein	–	–	x
Gelifex	Hydrogel	–	–	x
Hard devices				
Regain	Pyrolytic carbon	x	–	–
CL-Disc	Zirconia ceramic	x	–	–

nucleus replacement devices have been in development and until now various devices as shown below have been produced.

Types of nucleus replacement devices

Due to the rapid growth of technology there is a multiplicity of implants that are already in clinical use or under clinical trial. In principle, contained devices and devices with predefined geometry can be distinguished from uncontained or injectable devices (Table 1).

Contained and predefined devices

The Prosthetic Disc Nucleus PDN (Raymedica, Inc., Bloomington, Minnesota) assumes the cushioning function of a normal disc and simultaneously maintains disc height and flexibility. The device is composed of a hydrogel pellet that is surrounded by a polyethylene layer. The pellet absorbs water through which it is able to swell powerfully, restoring or maintaining disc height. The outer polyethylene fibers prevent unlimited swelling and minimize the horizontal spreading. This guarantees the maintenance of the implant shape even when overloading the spine. Each pellet has small platinum-iridium marker wires that are embedded in the hydrogel to visualize the position and orientation of the implants by fluoroscopy during surgery and by ordinary radiograph imaging after surgery [1]. Originally a two-pillow hydrogel, at present a single-pillow hydrogel, the new PDN-SOLO, is used (Fig. 1A, B).

The PDN has been a landmark for the development of nucleus replacement devices and is currently the device with the largest human clinical experience.

The NeuDisc (Replication Medical, Inc., New Brunswick, New Jersey) is another hydrogel device (Fig. 2A, B) that has been introduced recently in human trials. Similar to the PDN device it expands

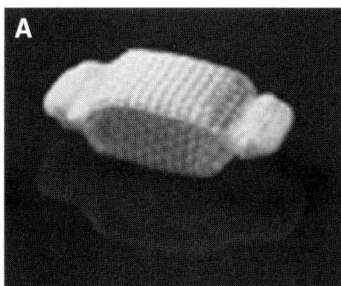

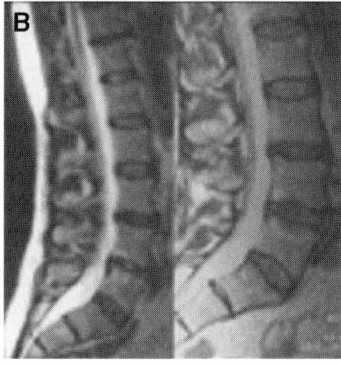

Fig. 1. (*A*) PDN-SOLO device. (*B*) MRI PDN-Dual (preoperative, postoperative).

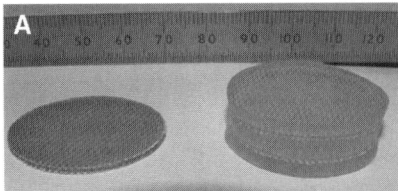
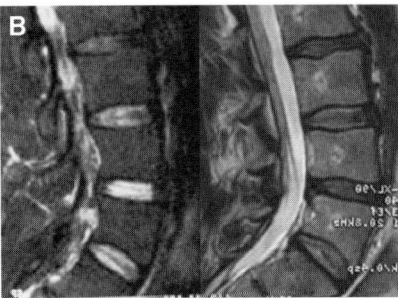

Fig. 2. (*A*) Neudisc device (preoperative, postoperative). (*B*) MRI Neudisc case.

preferentially in the axial direction by imbibing water. In contrast to the PDN the NeuDisc is not surrounded by an outer polyethylene jacket but by structured layers that are located inside the device. The proprietary hydrogel is characterized by excellent biostability, biocompatibility, and biomechanical properties and mimics the structural features of the nucleus pulposus [18].

The DASCOR (Disc Dynamics Inc., Eden Prairie, Minnesota) is a balloon device that will be filled with an injectable cool polyurethane polymer. The void is filled completely due to the fact that the polyurethane polymer is delivered under pressure [18]. The polyurethane polymer is contained due to the balloon. First clinical trials are under investigation.

Unconstrained devices

The Newcleus (Zimmer Spine, Warsaw, Indiana) is an unconstrained elastic memory coiling spiral made of polycarbonate urethane. The device functions as a spacer with some shock absorbing capability. First clinical trials started in Europe but the device is still under further development.

The Aquarelle (Stryker Corp., Kalamazoo, Michigan), a polyvinyl alcohol hydrogel nucleus replacement, has also undergone significant development and testing. Different from the PDN, the Aquarelle does not need a rehydration period postoperatively because it is implanted in a hydrated state. The device is viscoelastic and provides uniform pressure across the endplate. In opposite to the PDN device the lifting force is much less.

Injectable devices

An alternative to the devices mentioned previously are injectable substances that act more as a void filler.

The SINUX ANR (J&J DePuy, Raynham, Massachusetts) is a liquid polymethylsiloxane polymer that completely fills the void that is left from the removed nuclear material. It cures in approximately 15 minutes into a resilient elastic mass [18].

The BioDisc (Cryolife, Inc., Kennesaw, Georgia) is an injectable protein hydrogel device consisting of a mixture of serum albumin and gluteraldehyde.

The NuCore IDN (Spine Wave Inc., Shelton, Connecticut) is a protein polymer that is created through DNA bacterial synthesis fermentation. As protein polymers do not contain human or animal components, the risk for transmitting or causing diseases is reduced.

The Gelifex (Gelifex, Inc., Philadelphia, Pennsylvania) is a polymer that is liquid at room temperature and solidifies at body temperature.

In addition to these devices, devices made of memory metal stent, peak nucleus devices, and carbon-coated metal devices are under evaluation. None of these devices is in clinical use at present.

Indications

To achieve a high surgical success rate, careful patient selection is crucial. Among all of the currently used clinical study protocols for the different devices, the least common denominator are patients between 18 and 65 years old with degenerative disc disease, dominant low back pain, and back or leg pain who have failed conservative treatment. Because the failed nucleus will be replaced and will not be fixed into its position, a relatively intact annulus container with strong mechanical properties mustbe present. Therefore the disc height reduction should not exceed more than 50% of the original height.

In general, patients with osteoporosis, endplate problems, posterior element disorders (eg, stenosis, facit arthritis, isthmic pathologies), and infection tumors should be excluded.

For the longest used partial disc replacement device, the PDN, a disc height reduction of more

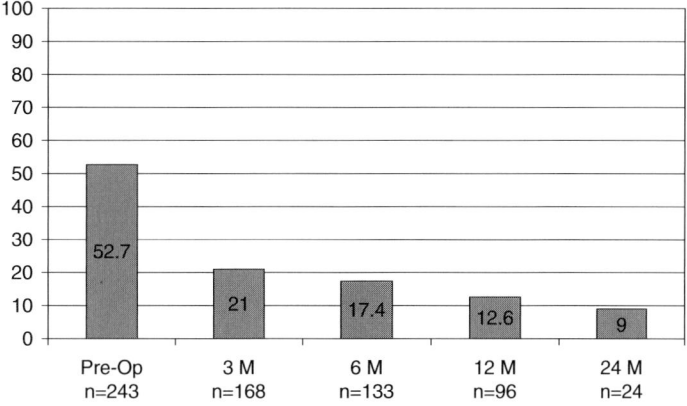

Fig. 3. Oswestry disability scores for patients with PDN device implantation, preoperative to 24 months.

than 50% and a BMI of 30 or greater have been analyzed as a reason for failures.

Results

Despite extensive information and use of implants, there are long-term studies only from the PDN device. The results of these German/Swedish and Korean studies are available as world data.

A worldwide clinical multicenter study with paired implants on 243 patients has shown marked improvement in pain levels.

The mean Oswestry score preoperative was 52.7. Postoperative the score dropped to 21 at the 3-months follow up, 17.4 at the 6-months follow up, and improved further to 12.6 after 12 months and 9.0 after 24 months (Fig. 3).

The VAS score declined similarly. The mean VAS score before surgery was 7.1, after 3 months 3.0, 6 months 3.0, 12 months 2.5, and it decreased to 1.8 after 24-months follow up (Fig. 4).

In addition, there was also an increase in disc height, which is a prerequisite for segmental stability to minimize nonphysiologic movements that may cause additional tearing of the annulus [19]. For 218 patients, the average disc height preoperative was 8.1 mm. It increased to 10.5 mm after 3 months, the 6 months follow up showed a disc height of 10.3 mm, the 12 months follow up 9.7 mm, and after 24 months the average disc height was 10.2 mm (Fig. 5).

The most common complications that have been reported for the use of PDN implantation are migration/extrusion as well as severe endplate reaction together with subsidence. The overall complication rate reduced from initially 53% to less than 25% due to improved implant design and surgical tech-

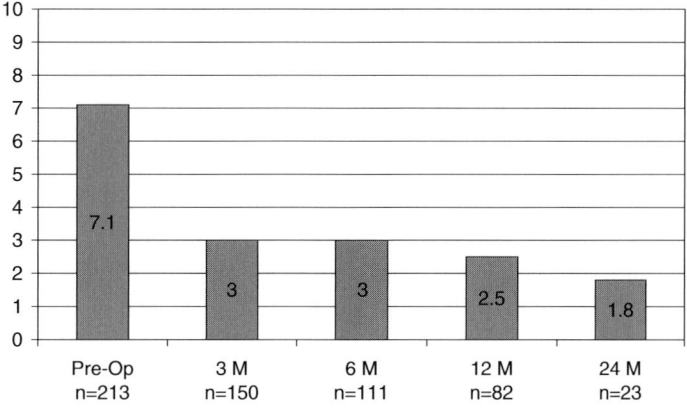

Fig. 4. Visual analog scale (VAS) for patients with PDN device implantation, preoperative to 24 months.

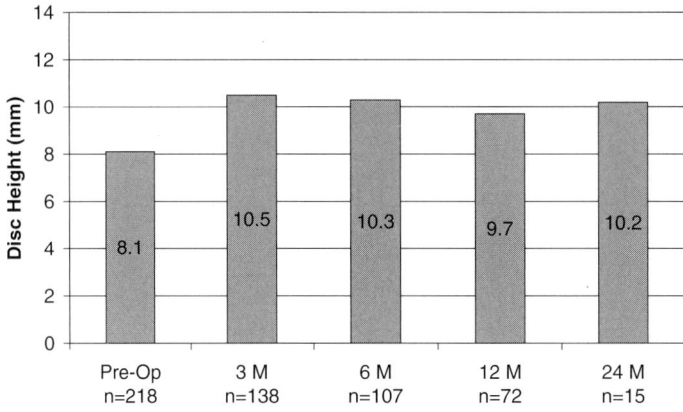

Fig. 5. Disc height before and after surgery.

niques. As a result of the not satisfying clinical outcome, the PDN-SOLO has been introduced. With the PDN-SOLO the overall complication rate could be reduced significantly and is now less than 10%. Also a suitable surgical approach can achieve a considerable reduction of the extrusion rate. By using the anterolateral transpsoatic approach (ALPA), the PDN extrusion could be completely reduced [20].

Summary

Up to now, no standards have been defined with regard to the degree of annulus degeneration and disc height loss up to which a nucleus implant can be successfully implanted.

The nucleus replacement is based on the assumption that the annulus and the endplates are still functioning properly [5]. These considerations have to be included in the patient selection and the indications for surgery. Reaction to the implant tissue interface can occur as well as other problems including wear and implant longevity problems, possible degradation processes within the nucleus material that might lead for re-intervention after 15 to 20 years, and the risk of herniation of the new, artificial nucleus. Therefore the current use of any of these devices should be investigated very precisely also in the near future and the patients should be selected very carefully following the criteria that have been defined in the known literature. Patients with risk factors like decreased bone density, increased BMI, or multilevel degeneration should be excluded. An optimal and careful surgical technique should be performed. Due to the rapidly growing number of new technologies in this field, a certain risk exists to lose the overview and to evaluate every single technique properly.

References

[1] Ray CD. The PDN® prosthetic disc nucleus device. Eur Spine J 2002;11(Suppl. 2):137–42.

[2] Cassidy JJ, Hiltner A, Baer E. Hierarchical structure of the intervertebral disc. Connect Tissue Res 1989;23: 75–88.

[3] Buckwalter JA. Aging and degeneration of the human intervertebral disc. Spine 1995;20:1307–14.

[4] Götz W, Barnert S, Bertagnoli R, et al. Immunhistchemical localisation of the small proteoglycans decorin and biglycan in human intervertebral discs. Cell Tissue Res 1997;289:185–90.

[5] Bao QB, Mc Cullen GM, Higham PA, et al. The artificial disc: theory, design and materials. Biomaterials 1996;17:1157–67.

[6] Studer A. Nucleus prosthesis: a new concept. Eur Spine J 2002;11(Suppl 2):154–6.

[7] Fennell AJ, Jones AP, Hukins DW. Migration of the nucleus pulposus within the intervertebral disc during flexion and extension of the spine. Spine 1996;21: 2753–7.

[8] Klein JA, Hickey DS, Hukins DW. Radial bulging of the annulus fibrosis during compression of the intervertebral disc. J Biomech 1983;16:211–7.

[9] Meakin JR, Redpath TW, Hukins DW. The effect of partial removal of the nucleus pulposus from the intervertebral disc on the response of the human annulus fibrosis to compression. Clin Biomech 2001; 16:121–8.

[10] Bertagnoli R. Disc surgery in motion. SpineLine 2004; 6:23–8.

[11] Wang ST, Goel VK, Fu CY, et al. Posterior instrumentation reduces differences in spine stability as a

[12] Ray CD. The artificial disc: introduction, history, and socioeconomics. In: Weinstein JN, editor. Clinical efficacy and outcome in the diagnosis and treatment of low back pain. New York: Raven Press; 1992. p. 205–25.
[13] Fernstrom V. Arthroplasty with intercorporal endoprosthesis in herniated disc and painful disc. Acta Chir Scand 1966;355(6):154–9.
[14] Hamby WB, Glaser HT. Replacement of spinal intervertebral discs with locally polymenting methyl methacrylate. J Neurosurg 1959;16:311–3.
[15] Nachemson AL. Some mechanical properties of the lumbar intervertebral disc. Bull Hosp Joint Dis 1962;23:130–2.
[16] Ambrosio L, DeSantis R, Nicolais L. Composite hydrogels for implants. Proc Inst Mech Engl 1998;212(2):93–9.
[17] Iatridis JC, Weidenbaum M, Seton LA, Mow VC. Is the nucleus pulposus a solid or a fluid? Mechanical behaviours of the nucleus pulposus of the human intervertebral disc. Spine 1996;21(10):1174–84.
[18] Viscogliosi AG, Viscogliosi JJ, Viscogliosi MR. Beyond total disc. The future of spine surgery. Spine Industry Analysis Series. New York: Viscogliosi Bros., LLC; May 2004. p. 131–98.
[19] Bertagnoli R, Schönmayr R. Surgical and clinical results with the PDN® prosthetic disc-nucleus device. Eur Spine J 2002;11(Suppl 2):143–8.
[20] Bertagnoli R, Vazquez RJ. The Anterolateral Trans-PsoaticApproach (ALPA): a new technique for implanting prosthetic disc-nucleus devices. J Spinal Disord Tech 2003;16(4):398–404.

result of different cage orientations: an in vitro study. Spine 2005;30(1):62–7.

Cervical Total Disc Replacement, Part I: Rationale, Biomechanics, and Implant Types

Mahidhar M. Durbhakula, MD[a], Gary Ghiselli, MD[b],*

[a]Department of Orthopaedic Surgery, Case Western Reserve University, 11100 Euclid Avenue, Cleveland, OH 44106, USA
[b]Denver Spine Center, 701 E. Hampden, Suite 120, Denver, CO 80113, USA

Anterior cervical discectomy and fusion (ACDF) remains the standard treatment for disc herniation and degenerative disc disease refractory to conservative treatment. Although effective in pain relief and decompression of neural elements, ACDF is associated with numerous complications including adjacent-segment degeneration, donor site morbidity, and pseudarthrosis. The success of joint arthroplasty and the adverse sequelae associated with fusion has stimulated research and development of artificial disc replacement. Although considerable progress has been made in the development of lumbar total disc replacement (TDR), developments in cervical TDR have been slower to emerge. The purpose of this article is to review the anatomy of the intervertebral disc and to discuss the rationale and implant types available for cervical TDR. Part 2 of this series reviews the results and complications of available cervical TDR prostheses.

Anatomy and pathophysiology

The cervical spine is composed of seven vertebral bodies with intervening intervertebral discs. These discs are critical for normal motion and biomechanics of the cervical spine. Discs function to provide load bearing and to optimize motion at intervertebral segments. The intervertebral disc is composed of an outer anulus fibrosis and a central nucleus pulposus, separated by a transitional zone. The anulus fibrosis is composed primarily of an organized network of type I collagen, contributing to the tensile strength of the disc. The nucleus pulposus is composed of water, proteoglycans, and type II collagen. The type II collagen is important in providing compressive strength, whereas the proteoglycan maintains water content and hydration in the nucleus pulposus.

Numerous investigators have compared the intervertebral disc to an inflated tire [1,2]. The air of the tire is analogous to the nucleus and transition zone. With pressure, forces are evenly distributed outward. The anulus is comparable to the tire itself, and the tensile strength from the anulus allows the anulus to resist stress from the nucleus. With aging, the nucleus loses water content and becomes more fibrous. As a result, the disc loses elasticity, resulting in the formation of clefts and fissures. The disc eventually collapses, the anulus bulges, and spur formation occurs at the anulus and uncovertebral joints. All of these factors contribute to pain and mechanical compression of neural structures.

Cervical end plates play an important role in bearing compressive load and preventing graft subsidence following ACDF, corpectomy, or TDR. Truumees et al [3] performed a cadaveric study of cervical end plates. Numerous factors including increasing age, female sex, decreased bone mineral density, caudal vertebral level, and aggressive end plate burring were noted to result in lower end plate fracture loads in compression. Other studies have investigated the regional strength of vertebral end plates. Lowe et al [4] conducted an in vitro study of thoracic and lumbar end plates and found that the

* Corresponding author.
E-mail address: g.g@denverspine.com (G. Ghiselli).

posterolateral end plate has the highest maximum load to failure. The central portion of the end plate provided the least resistance to subsidence. Complete removal of the end plate results in significant reduction in end plate strength, whereas partial end plate removal was shown to have adequate strength while providing a highly vascular bed for fusion.

Rationale for cervical total disc replacement

Treatment for herniated cervical discs in patients without neurologic deficit consists initially of nonoperative management consisting of anti-inflammatory medications, physical therapy, and epidural steroid injections in some cases. When conservative measures fail or when a neurologic deficit exists, surgical decompression is indicated.

Traditionally, ACDF has been performed for cases of cervical radiculopathy or myelopathy resulting from disc herniation. This technique involves anterior decompression of the disc space, followed by insertion of structural bone graft with or without anterior cervical plating and immobilization in a rigid cervical orthosis. Anterior cervical discectomy allows removal of the offending disc fragment, whereas fusion decreases pain associated with motion at the affected level and prevents progressive instability. Bohlman et al [5] followed patients treated with Robinson ACDF for treatment of cervical radiculopathy and found that ACDF was effective in relief of pain and resolution of neurologic symptoms.

Although fusion at single or multiple levels of the cervical spine allows for decompression of neural structures and restoration of disc height, it has been shown to alter the normal biomechanics of the cervical spine, leading to adjacent-segment degeneration. Hilibrand et al [6] followed 374 patients with Smith-Robinson anterior cervical fusion and found that 25.6% of patients had symptomatic adjacent-segment disease at 10-year follow-up. Incidence of adjacent-segment degeneration was higher at the C5-6 and C6-7 levels. Goffin et al [7] followed patients with anterior cervical arthrodesis and found a 92% incidence of adjacent-segment degeneration at 5-year follow-up.

Pseudarthrosis is another complication frequently associated with ACDF. Several studies have demonstrated a direct relationship between pseudarthrosis rate and number of levels fused. Brodke and Zdeblick [8] reported their results of ACDF using the modified Smith-Robinson technique. The fusion rate for single-level procedures was 97%, which decreased to 83% with fusion at three levels. Bohlman et al [5] reported an overall pseudarthrosis rate of 13% at an average 6-year follow-up. The rate of pseudarthrosis was 11% in single-level fusions and increased to 27% with multilevel fusions. Sixty-seven percent of patients with pseudarthrosis were symptomatic, with 17% requiring revision surgery.

Traditionally, autologous iliac crest bone graft has been used for ACDF procedures. Numerous donor site complications have been reported, including pain, infection, meralgia paresthetica and pelvic fracture, and neurovascular injury [9]. The overall complication rate for iliac crest harvest varies within the literature. Sandhu et al [10] reported a major complication rate of 1% to 25%, including deep infection, fracture, chronic pain, and herniation of abdominal contents. Minor complications such as superficial infection were reported to vary from 9% to 25%. The most frequent complication following bone graft harvest is chronic pain, with reports as high as 25% [11].

Cervical TDR has emerged as a promising alternative for the management of cervical disc herniation. The primary goals of cervical TDR are to remove the offending disc while restoring disc height and segment motion. Although never proved, motion preservation with TDR is intended to reduce adjacent-level disease. Similar to ACDF, TDR involves anterior decompression of the disc at the level of pathology. A cervical disc prosthesis is then inserted into the evacuated disc space in place of bone graft. Preservation of motion at the affected disc level restores normal biomechanics and offers several advantages. First, cervical TDR maintains normal cervical motion at the level of pathology. By preserving motion in the cervical spine, advanced adjacent-segment degeneration in avoided. Second, problems with graft incorporation and morbidity associated with iliac crest bone harvest are avoided. Finally, duration of postoperative immobilization is decreased in comparison to patients undergoing fusion procedures, which facilitates rapid return to normal activity.

Indications

Symptomatic cervical disc disease and herniation without neurologic deficit should initially be treated with a trial of nonoperative management. In fact, approximately 90% of symptomatic cervical disc disease responds to a combination of nonsteroidal anti-inflammatory drugs and physical therapy with traction. Cervical TDR provides an alternative to decompression and arthrodesis in patients with refractory disc disease in the cervical spine.

Inclusion criteria include symptomatic disc disease at only one level in the cervical spine. Single-level disease is a requirement in current trials of cervical TDR. If shown to be beneficial in single-level disease, application of TDR to multilevel disease would have a profound impact on preservation of cervical biomechanics and prevention of adjacent-segment disease. Other inclusion criteria include young patients (<60 years) with symptoms refractory to a thorough trial of conservative management.

Exclusion criteria for cervical TDR include pathology at more than one level, prior fusion at an adjacent level, instability on flexion–extension radiographs, and severe facet arthrosis at the affected level. History of prior cervical laminectomy and posterior compressive disease not amenable to decompression through an anterior approach are also contraindications to TDR. Other relative contraindications to cervical TDR include poor bone quality (ie, osteoporosis), infection, and rheumatoid arthritis.

Biomaterials and biomechanics

The goals of cervical TDR are to reproduce the normal motion of the cervical spine and to retain the normal biomechanical properties of the intervertebral disc. Because it is not possible to reproduce the exact biomechanical properties of native interverterbral disc, existing biomaterials represent a compromise of material strength and function. Materials that are commonly used in design include metals and polymers. Metals provide the necessary strength, ductility, and toughness needed for load bearing, whereas some polymers provide low-friction surfaces for articulation and "shock absorption."

Hallab et al [12] identified several criteria that are important for optimizing materials selection in TDR. These criteria include preservation of kinematics and biomechanics, preservation of intervertebral space, biocompatibility, revisability, and life expectancy of the materials used.

Hallab et al [12] studied the four materials that are most commonly used in cervical TDR: titanium alloys, cobalt alloys, stainless steels, and ultrahigh molecular weight polyethylene (UHMWPE). Titanium alloys possess the highest corrosion resistance and tissue compatibility, making titanium an attractive material for porous coatings of end plates in TDR. In addition, titanium allows for higher-quality postoperative imaging with MRI and CT scans. Cobalt alloys demonstrate good wear resistance, making them useful for articulation with UHMWPE surfaces. Stainless steel demonstrates good ductility but poor corrosion resistance. Finally, UHMWPE is useful for providing low-friction surfaces but raises concerns with wear debris. Cross-linking with gamma irradiation may help to improve wear resistance at the expense of fracture toughness, which may not be a worthwhile trade-off in the cervical spine. In addition, recent studies have questioned the shock absorption capability of polyethylene. LeHuec et al [13] compared the shock absorption capacity of lumbar TDR using a UHMWPE core versus a metal-on-metal design. No difference was noted between the two designs, demonstrating the limited shock absorbing capacity of polyethylene.

At this time, the ideal materials are unknown. Metal-on-metal designs may reduce osteolysis, although this has not yet been observed following TDR. Titanium-on-titanium has historically been a poor bearing surface. Titanium-UHMWPE has been shown to be a poor bearing surface in total hip prostheses, but this has not been a problem with the ProDisc Cervical-C implant (Synthes-Stratec, Oberdorf, Switzerland) [14]. Numerous trials comparing TDR designs with different biomaterial composition should help define the ideal characteristics and properties of cervical TDR.

The biomechanics of cervical TDR are complex due to coupled motions of the uncovertebral, intervertebral, and facet joints. Advances in understanding of the cervical spine biomechanics have facilitated design of cervical TDR systems. The basic biomechanical goal is to preserve motion and reduce adjacent-level disease. Quantity of angular motion in the sagittal and coronal planes is likely to provide protection against adjacent-segment disease. Also important is the quality of motion, including radius of curvature, shear properties, and location of the instantaneous axis of rotation. The quality of motion in TDR is critical because the facets have highly conforming anatomy and play a large role in dictating the instantaneous axis of rotation. Nonanatomic motion in cervical TDR may result in progressive facet arthrosis and pain. In addition, constraint may be important in facet preservation. Huang et al [15] described the role of constraint in lumbar TDR. Unconstrained designs provide a physiologic mobile instantaneous axis of rotation and increased range of motion and may prevent excessive facet joint forces with motion. Constrained designs were shown to protect the posterior elements from shear loading, which may be important due to the considerable shear loads with activities of daily living. Clearly, it is not possible to perfectly replicate the kinematics of a healthy motion segment. Ongoing studies will help to define the ideal biomechanical configuration of TDR designs in the cervical spine.

Cervical total disc replacement implant types

Over the past 40 years, there have been several designs for cervical disc prosthesis. Current systems for TDR in the cervical spine use different materials and geometric configurations. Metal-on-metal prostheses include the Bristol Disc, the Cummins design, and the Prestige Disc (Medtronic Sofamor Danek, Memphis, Tennessee), and the Cervicore (SpineCore, Stryker Spine, Allendale, New Jersey) system. Another commonly used design uses metal end plates with a "plastic" center. Prostheses using a polyethylene center include the ProDisc-C (Synthes-Stratec) and the Porous-Coated Motion (PCM) cervical artificial disc (Cervitech, Inc., Rockaway, New Jersey). The Bryan Cervical Disc Prosthesis (Medtronic Sofamor Danek, Memphis, Tennessee) is another metal-polymer implant that uses a polyurethane center.

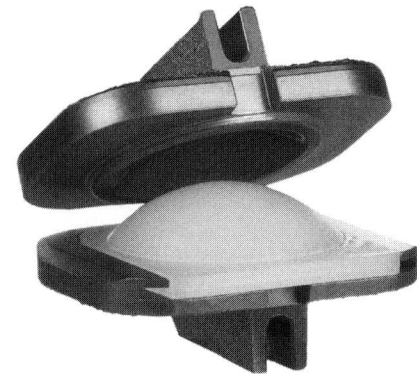

Fig. 2. The ProDisc-C implant. (*Courtesy of* Synthes-Stratec, Oberdorf, Switzerland, with permission.)

Metal-on-metal designs

The original metal-on-metal design for cervical TDR was the Cummins design, which used type-316 stainless steel in a ball-and-socket articulation to allow apparent translation. Fixation is achieved with titanium screws placed anteriorly in the vertebral body. Additional stability is achieved through compression of vertebral bodies against ridges in the metal prosthesis.

The next generation of metal-on-metal prosthesis was the Bristol Disc, which modified the Cummin's disc to a ball-and-trough articulation to allow for more physiologic translation at the level of replacement. Finally, the Prestige Disc uses a similar design to the Bristol Disc but has a lower profile and improved instrumentation to allow for easier implantation.

The Prestige Disc (Medtronic Sofamor Danek) uses stainless steel in a metal-on-metal configuration (Fig. 1). Although metal-on-metal designs are associated with potential for metal debris and increased systemic concentrations of metal ions, the purpose of this design is to avoid the increased particulate wear debris found in metal-polymer designs.

Metal-polymer designs

The Prodisc-C prosthesis uses a cobalt-chrome alloy for the end plates and UHMWPE as a central polymer (Fig. 2). The cobalt-chrome end plates are coated with titanium plasmapore for tissue com-

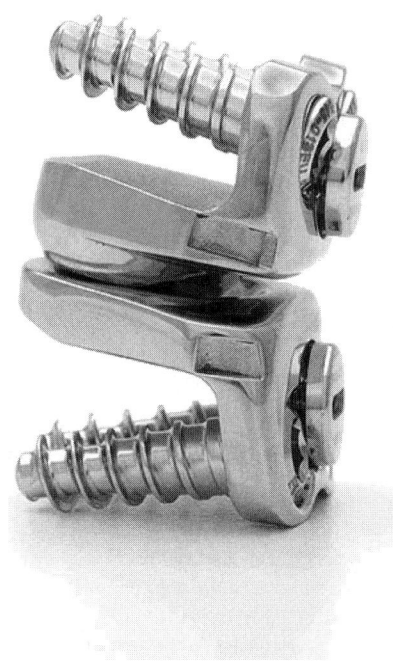

Fig. 1. The Prestige disc. (*Courtesy of* Medtronic Sofamor Danek, Memphis, Tennessee, with permission.)

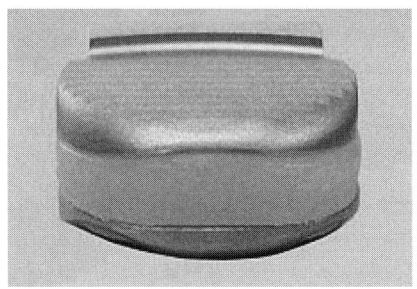

Fig. 3. The PCM prosthesis. (*Courtesy of* Cervitech, Inc., Rockaway, New Jersey, with permission.)

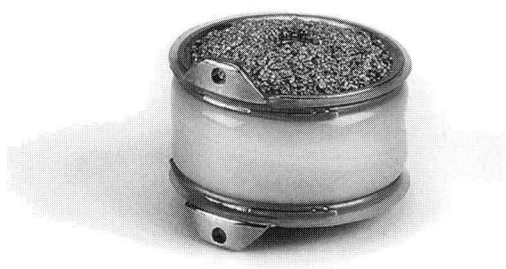

Fig. 4. The Bryan Disc. (*Courtesy of* Medtronic Sofamor Danek, Memphis, Tennessee, with permission.)

patibility and bone ingrowth. A locking core of UHMWPE provides a ball-and-socket articulation.

The PCM prosthesis uses a large-radius UHMWPE core with cobalt-chrome end plates that allow for bone ingrowth (Fig. 3). Biomechanical studies have identified the role of the posterior longitudinal ligament in stability of the cervical spine following anterior cervical discectomy [16]. The PCM prosthesis accounts for integrity of the posterior longitudinal ligament with low-profile and fixed designs. The low-profile PCM implant is used in cases in which the posterior longitudinal ligament is preserved. If the posterior longitudinal ligament has to be removed as part of the spinal cord decompression, then a fixed PCM prosthesis is preferred. The fixed implant incorporates anterior flanges and screws to enhance stability of the construct.

The Bryan Disc (Medtronic Sofamor Danek) attempts to preserve normal kinematics by using an axially symmetric prosthesis to mimic normal flexion, extension, and lateral bending. This prosthesis uses porous-coated, clamshell-shaped titanium end plates with a polycarbonate polyurethane core (Fig. 4). A unique feature of the Bryan Disc is a polyurethane membrane that surrounds the articulation to reduce friction and contain debris. In vitro studies have confirmed favorable wear characteristics of the Bryan Disc prosthesis [17–28].

Summary

Cervical TDR is an attractive alternate to arthrodesis for management of disc degeneration and herniation in the cervical spine. Theoretic advantages of TDR include preservation of normal motion and biomechanics in the cervical spine and reduction of adjacent-segment degeneration. Other potential advantages include faster return to normal activity and elimination of the need for bone graft and associated donor site morbidity.

This article introduces the rationale and various implant types available for cervical TDR. Part 2 of this series reviews the results and complications of specific implant designs.

References

[1] Huang RC, Sandhu HS. The current status of lumbar total disc replacement. Orthop Clinics N Am 2004; 35(1):33–42.

[2] Diwan AD, Parvataneni HK, Khan SN, et al. Current concepts in intervertebral disk restoration. Orthop Clin N Am 2000;31(3):453–64.

[3] Truumees E, Demetropoulos CK, Yang KH, et al. Failure of human cervical endplates: a cadaveric experimental model. Spine 2003;28(19):2204–8.

[4] Lowe TG, Hashim S, Wilson LA, et al. A biomechanical study of regional endplate strength and cage morphology as it relates to structural interbody support. Spine 2004;29(21):2389–94.

[5] Bohlman HH, Emery SE, Goodfellow DB, et al. Robinson anterior cervical discectomy and arthrodesis for cervical radiculopathy. Long-term follow-up of one hundred and twenty-two patients. J Bone Joint Surg [Am] 1993;75(9):1298–307.

[6] Hilibrand AS, Carlson GD, Palumbo MA, Jones PK, Bohlman HH. Radiculopathy and myelopathy at segments adjacent to the site of a previous anterior cervical arthrodesis. J Bone Joint Surg [Am] 1999;81(4): 519–28.

[7] Goffin J, Geusens E, Vantomme N, et al. Long term follow-up after interbody fusion at cervical spine. J Spinal Disord Tech 2004;17(2):79–85.

[8] Brodke DS, Zdeblick TA. Modified Smith-Robinson procedure for anterior cervical discectomy and fusion. Spine 1992;17:S427–30.

[9] Brown CA, Eismont FJ. Complications in spinal fusion. Orthop Clinics N Am 1998;29(4):679–99.

[10] Sandhu HS, Grewal HS, Parvataneni H. Bone grafting for spinal fusion. Orthop Clinics N Am 1999;30(4): 685–98.

[11] Summers BN, Eisenstein SM. Donor site pain from the ilium: a complication of lumbar spine fusion. J Bone Joint Surg Br 1989;71:677–80.

[12] Hallab N, Link HD, McAfee PC. Biomaterial optimization in total disc arthroplasty. Spine 2003;28(205): S139–52.

[13] LeHuec JC, Kiaer T, Friesem T, et al. Shock absorption in lumbar disc prosthesis: a preliminary mechanical study. J Spinal Disord Tech 2003;16(4):346–51.

[14] Tropiano, et al. J Bone Joint Surg Am 2005, in press.

[15] Huang RC, Girardi FP, Cammisa FP, et al. The implications of constraint in lumbar total disc replacement. Spine 2003;28:412–7.

[16] McAfee PC, Cunningham B, Dmitriev A, et al.

Cervical disc replacement—Porous Coated Motion prosthesis: a comparative biomechanical analysis showing the key role of the posterior longitudinal ligament. Spine 2003;28(205):S176–85.

[17] Anderson PA, Rouleau JP, Bryan VE, et al. Wear analysis of the Bryan Cervical Disc prosthesis. Spine 2003;28(20):S186–94.

[18] Arrington ED, Smith WJ, Chambers HG, et al. Complications of iliac crest bone graft harvesting. Clin Orthop 1996;329:300–9.

[19] Boden SD, Balderston RA, Heller JG, et al. Disc replacements: this time will we really cure low-back and neck pain? J Bone Joint Surg Am 2004;86(2): 411–22.

[20] Bryan VE. Cervical motion segment replacement. Eur Spine J 2002;11:S92–7.

[21] Cummings BH, Robertson JT, Gill SS. Surgical experience with an implanted artificial cervical joint. J Neurosurg 1998;88:943–8.

[22] Emery SE, Fisher RS, Bohlman HH. Three-level anterior cervical discectomy and fusion: rRadiographic and clinical results. Spine 1997;22:2622–5.

[23] Goulet JA, Senunas LE, DeSilva GL, et al. Autogenous iliac crest bone graft: complications and functional assessment. Clin Orthop 1997;339:76–81.

[24] Guyer RD, Ohnmeiss DD. Intervertebral disc prostheses. Spine 2003;28(Suppl 15):S15–23.

[25] Hu RW, Bohlman HH. Fracture at the iliac bone graft harvest site after fusion of the spine. Clin Orthop 1994; 309:208–13.

[26] Sekhon L. Cervical arthroplasty in the management of spondylotic myelopathy. J Spinal Disord Tech 2003; 16(4):307–13.

[27] Wigfield CC, Gill SS, Nelson RJ, et al. The new Frenchay artificial cervical joint. Spine 2002;27(22): 2446–52.

[28] Zdeblick TA, Hughes SS, Riew KD, et al. Failed anterior cervical discectomy and arthrodesis. Analysis and treatment of thirty-five patients. J Bone Joint Surg [Am] 1997;79(4):523–32.

Cervical Total Disc Replacement, Part Two: Clinical Results

Rudolf Bertagnoli, MD[a,*], Neil Duggal, MD[b], Gwynedd E. Pickett, MD[b], Crispin C. Wigfield, MD[c], Steven S. Gill, MS[d], Armin Karg[e], Sandra Voigt[e]

[a]*Spine Center, St.-Elisabeth-Klinikum, St.-Elisabeth-Str. 23, 94315 Straubing, Germany*
[b]*Department of Clinical Neurological Sciences, London Health Sciences Center, The University of Western Ontario, 339 Windermere Road, London, ON N6A 5A5, Canada*
[c]*Spinal Research Unit, Department of Neurosurgery, Frenchay Hospital, Frenchay Park Road, Bristol BS16 1LE, UK*
[d]*Institute of Clinical Neuroscience, Department of Neurosurgery, Frenchay Hospital, Frenchay Park Road, Bristol BS16 1LE, UK*
[e]*Spine Center Straubing, Obere Bachstrasse 30 a, 94315 Straubing, Germany*

Variations on discectomy and fusion with autologous bone have been attempted with varying success. Successful orthopedic treatment of arthropathies, initially with large joint replacement and more recently with smaller joint replacements, has resulted in a heightened interest in spinal total disc replacement (TDR). Closer attention is being paid to the longer-term effects of spinal fusion, and an increasingly critical approach to assessing short- and long-term surgical outcome is being addressed. A cervical disc replacement should not adversely affect the associated facet joints, adjacent motion segments of the spine, and most important, the neurovascular elements of the spine. The cervical TDR implants with the most extensive clinical experience are the ProDisc-C (Synthes, Oberdorf, Switzerland), the Bryan Cervical Disc (Medtronic Sofamor Danek, Memphis, Tennessee), and the Bristol Disc (Medtronic Sofamor Danek, Memphis, Tennessee).

ProDisc-C

Design

The ProDisc-C prosthesis (Fig. 1) was designed to be implanted in a simple surgical procedure with a few steps. The ProDisc-C restores segmental motion, foraminal height, dynamic function, spinal balance, and stability of the cervical spine. The prosthesis consists of a modular design, two metal plates, and a polyethylene inlay that is safely secured into the lower end plate (snap mechanism). The metal end plates have a keel design for enhanced primary stability and fixation, and the end plate coverage with titanium plasma spray coating allows bony ingrowth and long-term fixation. The polyethylene inlay determines the height of the prosthesis. The prosthesis is designed for en bloc implantation.

Indications

Ideal patients for cervical TDR present with degenerative disc disease that has failed extensive nonsurgical treatment and is causing combinations of neck pain, myelopathy, and radiculopathy. Cervical TDR in patients with degenerative disease and isolated neck pain without neural compression symptoms is not yet recommended until more clinical data are available. There are several factors that exclude patients from being eligible to have this procedure, such as osteoporosis and osteopenia or other bone metabolic diseases, posterior facet arthropathy, severe myelopathy due to posterior vertebral body spinal cord compression, chronic infections, tumor, metabolic or systemic disease, or pertinent metallic allergies.

* Corresponding author.
  E-mail address: bertagnoli@pro-spine.com
  (R. Bertagnoli).

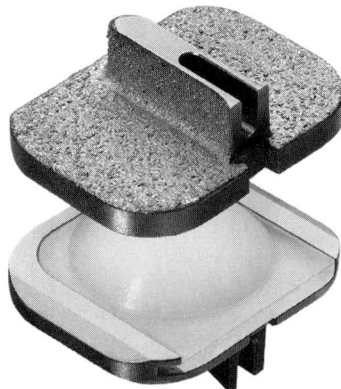

Fig. 1. Illustration of the ProDisc-C. (Courtesy of Synthes, Oberdorf, Switzerland from the surgical technique ProDisc-C © Stratec Medical 2005, Switzerland; with permission.)

Surgical approach

Before surgery, a complete clinical and radiographic assessment must be performed. The patient is situated in a supine position on a fluoroscopic imaging table to allow imaging in anteroposterior (AP) and lateral planes to locate the level of the diseased disc and to control the different surgical steps of the application. The anterior cervical spine is exposed using a standard-approach, standard retractor system or with the assistance of a specialized anterior spinal retractor system, the Cervical SynFrame (Synthes Spine, Oberdorf, Switzerland). After determining the midline, self-tapping retainer pins are fixed into the vertebral bodies. After application of the retainer, the discectomy is performed and distraction is performed with the distraction forceps. The retainer is adjusted to the distraction forceps accordingly, and the disc-extruded material and the cartilaginous end plates are removed. With a high-speed bur, the anterior and posterior part of the end plate is remodeled into a relatively flat surface. At least 60% to 70% of the natural end plate must be maintained.

After the end plate preparation is completed, specially designed trials that correspond to the height and AP diameter of the sizes available for the ProDisc-C are used to assess sizing under lateral fluoroscopy. After the appropriate size is determined, positioning along the midline is confirmed by AP fluoroscopy. Keel cuts are made using the prosthesis trial as the guide and a keel-cutting chisel. The trial and chisel are removed. Under lateral fluoroscopy, the prosthesis is inserted to an adequate depth. AP and

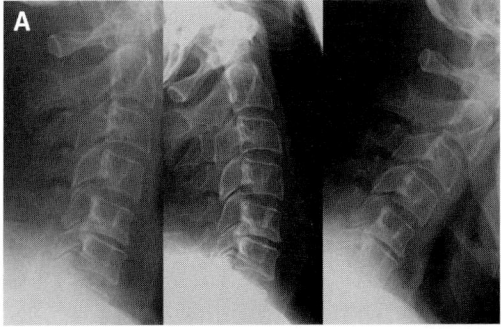

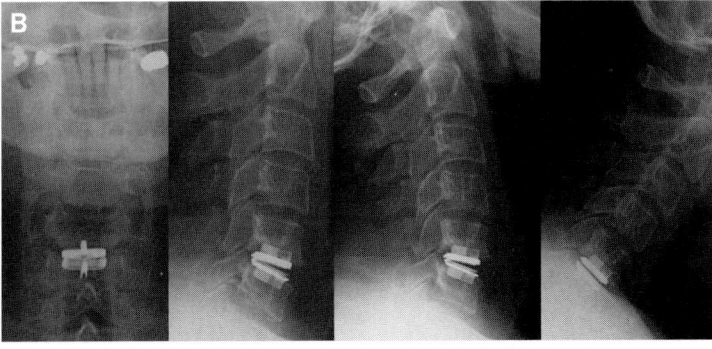

Fig. 2. (*A*) Preoperative radiographs (lateral, flexion, extension). (*B*) Postoperative radiographs (AP, lateral, flexion, extension).

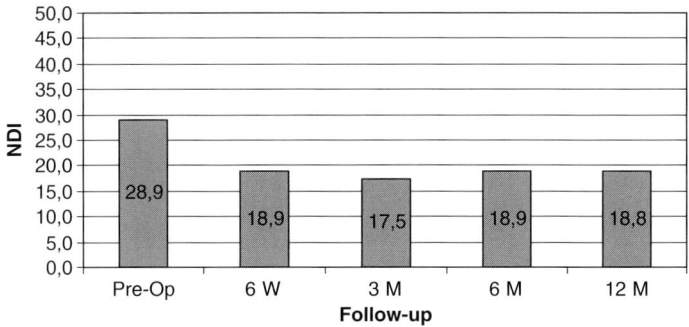

Fig. 3. Preoperative to 12-month follow-up NDI scores for patients with ProDisc-C implantation.

Results

In this study, only patients who had one level of cervical degenerative disc disease were surgically treated with a Prodisc-C implant. Twenty-seven patients with 1-year follow-up were included.

Patients were assessed preoperatively and postoperatively at 3 and 6 weeks and at 3, 6, and 12 months. The primary functional outcomes assessed pre- and postoperatively were disability and pain scores using the Neck Disability Index (NDI) and visual analog scale (VAS) scores. Additional clinical parameters included analysis of pre- and postoperative patient satisfaction, general neck pain, radicular pain, medication usage, and complications.

Pre- and postoperative radiographs (Fig. 2) were obtained in all patients, including AP, lateral, flexion, extension, and lateral bending films. Independent reviewers assessed radiographs for device-related loosening, dislodgment, or subsidence.

lateral fluoroscopy confirm appropriate placement. The incision is closed, completing the procedure.

The average age of the patients was 49 years (range, 31–66 years) at the time of surgery. Of the 27 patients, 13 were men and 14 were women. Three patients had prior surgery. Most cases were at the operative level of C5-6 (16 patients) and the remaining patients had surgery at C4-5 (2 patients) and C6-7 (9 patients).

The clinical outcome measures (Figs. 3–5) show sustained improvement at 1-year follow-up. The NDI scores show a 35% decrease at 6 weeks postoperatively that steadily continue to 1-year follow-up. Similarly, VAS scores drop 44% by 6 weeks postoperatively and remain constant. Range of motion (ROM) showed a 240% improvement at 1-year follow-up in comparison to the preoperative condition, and more important, ROM returned to a normal functional level of motion at about 10°.

Pain intensity and frequency was assessed in the neck and arms. The frequency and intensity of neck pain decreased similarly from the preoperative assessment by approximately 40%. In the arms, pain frequency and intensity resolved to less than half of the original value.

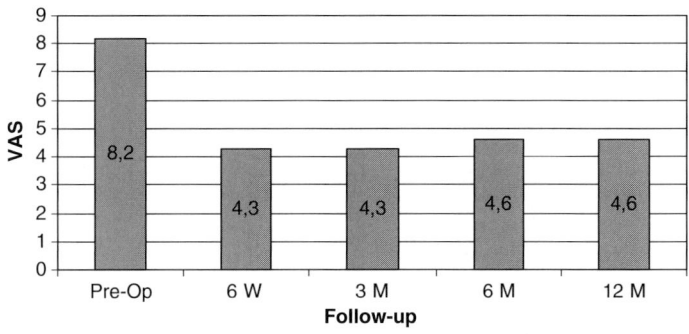

Fig. 4. Preoperative to 12-month follow-up VAS scores for patients with ProDisc-C implantation.

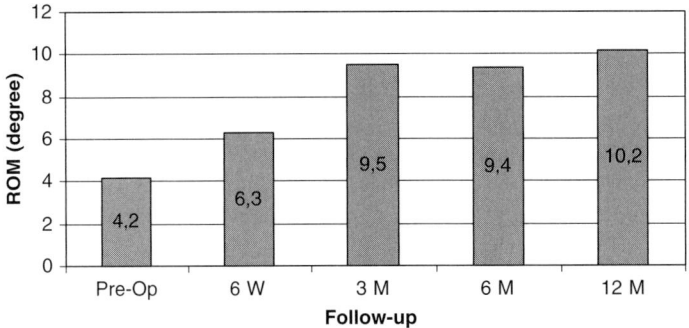

Fig. 5. Range of motion, preoperative to 12-month follow-up.

Patient satisfaction levels at 1-year follow-up were completely satisfied (52%), satisfied (36%), and not satisfied (12%). More patients initially reported being completely satisfied, but this rate dropped by approximately 20% over the first year. The percentage of patients who reported being satisfied rose during the year of follow-up by approximately 10%. At 3-week follow-up, none of the patients reported being not satisfied, but the percentage increased during follow-up.

There were no device-related complications in this study. The authors recorded no cases of loosening, subsidence, migration, metallic or polyethylene failure, allergic rejection/reaction, visceral or neurologic injuries caused by the implant components, or infection. There were no approach-related complications such as intraoperative fractures, hematomas, dural tears/leaks, postoperative airway compromise, esophageal or tracheal disruption, laryngeal nerve injury, or sympathetic nerve dysfunction. The authors observed no spontaneous fusions at the affected or adjacent levels.

Discussion

Because many of the new designs have the potential to become a standard of practice in medical care of degenerative disc disease, it becomes imperative to understand the biomechanical environment of the cervical spine and how each design works within that environment. Although well-controlled prospective, randomized studies are currently underway and provide excellent short-term data, long-term results truly show the advantage of arthroplasty over arthrodesis. This short series offers a glimpse into the clinical basis for arthroplasty and elucidates the lack of complications and short-term issues with cervical arthroplasty. It is hoped that long-term data will support the theory that arthroplasty reduces the incidence of adjacent-level disease because it restores functional motion, thereby maintaining normal loads at the adjacent levels.

Bryan Cervical Disc

Design

The Bryan Cervical Disc prosthesis consists of a low-friction polyurethane nucleus surrounded by a polyurethane sheath and situated between two titanium alloy shells. The biarticulating metal-on-polymer disc possesses elasticity and little compressibility and allows for unconstrained motion and translation through normal ROM. The prosthesis is axially symmetric, allowing for similar ROM in sagittal plane motion and in lateral bending.

Axial rotation of the Bryan disc is unconstrained. Preliminary biomechanical studies suggest a mobile center of rotation [1], allowing the device to accommodate a range of preoperative center-of-rotation values without subjecting the facets and ligaments to abnormal stresses. Abnormal shifting of the center of rotation following spinal arthroplasty has been implicated in recent reports of facet pain associated with prosthesis positioning [2].

Clinical results

Goffin et al [3] provided the first report of a large clinical series of patients treated with the Bryan Cervical Disc prosthesis. This multicenter, prospective cohort described preliminary results with insertion of the disc following anterior cervical discectomy for single-level degenerative disease. Patients with radiculopathy or myelopathy were recruited for the study. Although the investigators described 97 patients undergoing implantation with the device, clinical outcome data were reported for only 60 patients, with 30 reaching the 1-year postoperative end point. The outcome tools that were used included the Cervical Spine Research Society Assessment Scale and Short Form–36 (SF-36); results were reported using modified Odom's criteria. Success, defined by the investigators as excellent, good, or fair, was reported in 86% of patients at 6 months and 90% at 1 year. These promising clinical outcomes, however, are a result of the adequacy of neural decompression and are independent of the prosthesis. Perhaps more important, preserved ROM at the site of surgery was reported in 93% of patients at 6 months and in 88% at 1 year. No device failures, subsidence, or explantations were described. Device migration was detected in 1 patient and suspected in a another. This migration was attributed to incomplete milling of the end plates. Approach-related complications were also described [3].

A follow-up study by Goffin et al [4] reported longer follow-up on the single-level group and early clinical results with two-level implantation of the Bryan Cervical Disc. ROM analysis demonstrated preserved sagittal plane motion in 88% of single-level and 86% of two-level patients at 1 year, whereas clinical outcomes were rated as excellent, good, or fair in over 90% of patients (n = 89) at 1 year [4]. More recently, follow-up on this group of patients showed that 45 of 73 (62%) single-level patients with 2-year follow-up had "excellent" outcome, with 7 patients scored as good, 13 as fair, and 8 as poor [5]. SF-36 physical and mental component summary scores were significantly improved by 3 months postoperatively, and this improvement was maintained up to 2 years. Sagittal plane motion equal to or greater than 2° remained present in 88% of patients at 2 years [5]. Similarly encouraging results were reported for the two-level cohort, with 21 of 30 (70%) patients with 1-year follow-up outcome scored as excellent, 3 scored as good, 5 as fair, and 1 as poor. SF-36 scores again improved postoperatively, although the statistical significance was not reported [5].

A smaller prospective cohort confirmed preservation of motion and significant improvement in standardized clinical outcome tools including the NDI and SF-36. In this study, Duggal et al [6] also compared outcomes in patients suffering from soft disc herniations with those patients with spondylotic ridging causing foraminal stenosis. No statistically significant difference was found with respect to outcome scores between the two groups. In addition, when outcomes in patients undergoing arthroplasty for myelopathy were compared with patients who had radiculopathy, no difference in outcome or complication rate was found.

A functional disc prosthesis, which adequately mimics the in vivo function and biomechanics of an intervertebral disc, may be able to restore the functional spine unit and prevent subsequent adjacent segment degeneration. The authors recently assessed the in vivo kinematics of the Bryan artificial disc in a

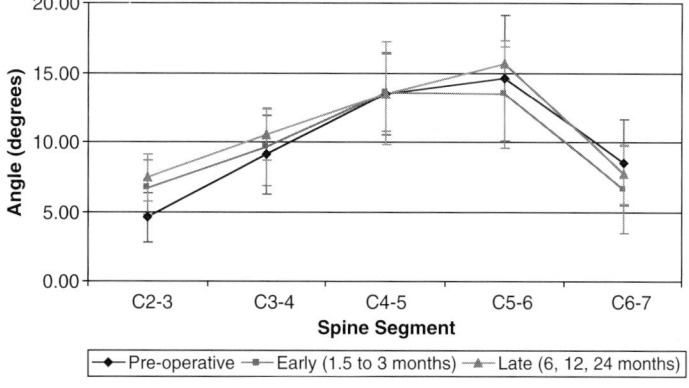

Fig. 6. Sagittal rotation for patients with a single C6/C7 prosthesis. The relative contribution of each spinal segment to global spinal motion did not change significantly following arthroplasty.

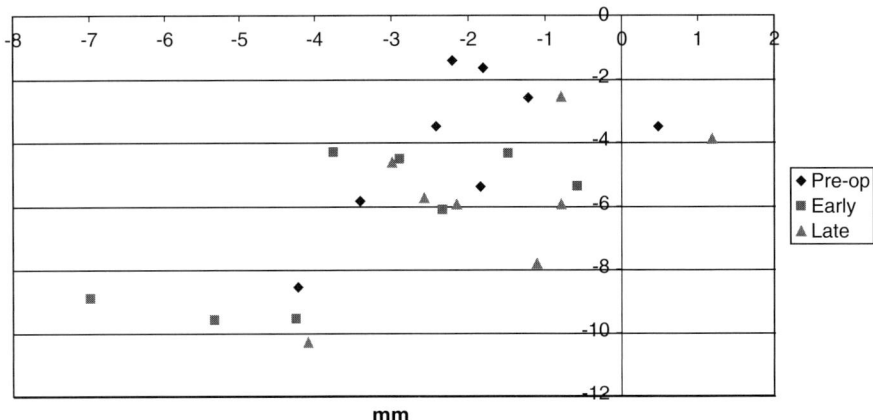

Fig. 7. C5-6 COR for patients with single C5-6 prosthesis. Preoperative center-of-rotation values (COR) plotted in (x,y) pairs show wide variability. The prosthesis was able to accommodate a similar range postoperatively, with no significant change in the distribution of the center-of-rotation locations.

prospectively enrolled cohort of 20 patients (24 discs) using quantitative motion analysis software to analyze intervertebral motion. Sagittal ROM, centers of rotation, horizontal translation, and disc height were not significantly altered following disc replacement compared with the preoperative state. The relative contribution of each spinal segment to sagittal rotation was preserved (Fig. 6).

The center of rotation at the level of surgery and at the adjacent levels was also preserved following arthroplasty (Fig. 7) [1].

These results suggest that the Bryan Cervical Disc replacement can preserve the preoperative kinematics of the cervical spine.

Complications

Complications reported following insertion of any cervical prosthesis may be divided into those specific to the prosthesis and those associated with anterior cervical discectomy [7,8]. Cerebrospinal fluid leak, esophageal injury, and wound hematomas were reported in the European studies, with an overall complication rate of 6.3% per operated level [4]. Inadequate neural decompression requiring repeat surgery was reported in 3 of 146 cases. Reported complications specific to the Bryan Cervical Disc, however, include anterior and posterior migration, end plate kyphosis, and failure to maintain motion [4,9]. The unconstrained nature of the disc has resulted in cases of worsened cervical kyphosis when implanted in patients with straight or kyphotic cervical curvatures, particularly those with a preoperative focal kyphosis at the operated segment [10]. No cases of subsidence or device failures have so far been reported in over 5500 implants worldwide [5].

Bristol Disc

Evolution

In the late 1980s, Brian Cummins, a neurosurgeon at Frenchay Hospital (Bristol, United Kingdom) tried to address the problem of maintaining motion in the cervical spine following surgery by introducing a simple ball-and-socket type of cervical joint. It was made out of type-316 stainless steel and had an upper hemispherical component that sat in a reciprocating lower cup, the two components secured to their respective vertebrae by means of anterior flanges and screws. In the first clinical trial, however, problems encountered included joint subluxation, screw pullouts, and screw fractures. The Cummins joint was redesigned by Gill to allow more physiologic motion to occur. Translation and rotation was achieved with the upper vertebral component being permitted to passively find its own axis of rotation as determined by the facet joints and coupled motion of adjacent vertebrae. The lower vertebral component had a shallow elliptic concavity rather than a reciprocating concave hemisphere on which the upper component could glide with point contact. In addition, the screw locking mechanism was redesigned to incorporate the Orion locking system (Medtronic Sofamor Danek). The overall bulk of the construct

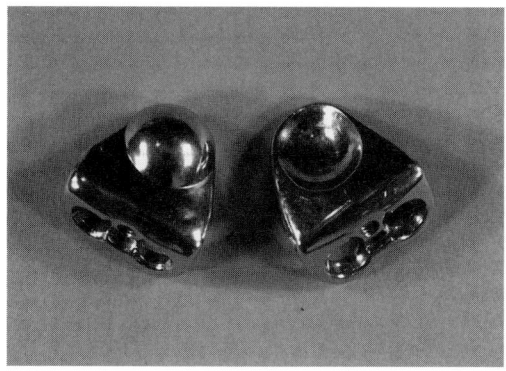

Fig. 8. Illustration of the two articulating components of the Bristol Disc without bone screws or locking screws. The lower component with the ellipsoid saucer is on the right.

was reduced. This new device was referred to as the Bristol Disc (Fig. 8).

The Bristol Disc pilot study

The aim of the pilot study was to assess the safety of the surgical technique, to closely monitor patients receiving the joint for evidence of adverse events, and to evaluate the clinical stability of the device and the ability of the implant to preserve segmental motion in the cervical spine. Secondary outcome measures of pain scores for neck and arm pain, myelopathy scores, and SF-36 scores were also assessed.

Joints were inserted between C3-4 and C6-7. No postoperative wound or periprosthetic infections were encountered. Motion was preserved and ranged between 3° and 12° (mean, 6.5°) at 2 years (Fig. 9'). Translation in an AP direction of up to 2 mm was achieved. All the joints stayed in place in the intervertebral space and there was no incidence of joint dislocation. Comparing data at 24 months with preoperative data from the questionnaires indicated improvement in all aspects of patient function and quality of life.

No changes in any of the categories of assessment reached statistical significance due to the small number of patients in this pilot study. Employment status improved. CT myelograms were performed on 4 patients and gave excellent imaging. None of the patients with CT myelograms demonstrated any neural compromise associated with the prosthesis. One patient had the joint removed after 12 months but her symptoms remained unchanged despite achieving a stable interbody fusion. Motion of the joint was maintained in all the remaining 14 patients at 24 months. Good stability of the prosthesis was demonstrated in all 14 patients with the device at 24 months.

It was necessary to be cautious of attaching too much significance to data arising from the questionnaires completed in this study. Most of the patients had a chronic history of neck disability punctuated by several previous interventions by a variety of clinicians. Some patients had taken part in pain management programs with limited success over preceding years. Hence, although the study entry criteria were strict, a far-from-homogeneous cohort was involved in this study. It was considered essential to gain as much information as possible about this device even if the small numbers involved made data interpretation limited. This study demonstrated that a prosthetic cervical joint that permits normal cervical spinal kinematics of rotation, angulation, and translation could be safely inserted. The study did not demonstrate any adverse effect occurring at adjacent vertebral levels [11].

Refined designs and improved clinical trials

During the initial pilot study, the Bristol Disc was renamed Prestige (Medtronic Sofamor Danek). Design modifications resulted in a reduced-profile product with bone ingrowth surfaces and a range of sizes (12 or 14 mm AP dimension with heights of 6 or 8 mm). The new discs were named Prestige II. The limitations of the pilot study called for more controlled clinical studies.

A multicenter, prospective, randomized controlled study was conducted. Four centers, from the United Kingdom, Belgium, Switzerland, and Australia, were involved. Fifty-five patients were enrolled in the study, with 27 receiving the Prestige II disc and 28 receiving fusion. Patients were eligible only if their sole diagnosis was degenerative disc disease affecting a single cervical intervertebral disc between

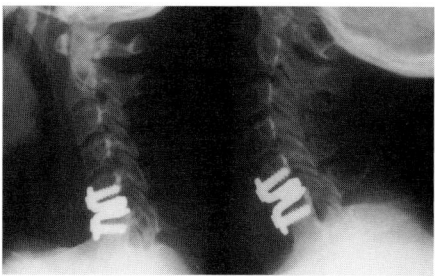

Fig. 9. Flexion (*left*) and extension (*right*) radiographs showing the degree of angulation achieved by the Bristol Disc (in this case, a total of 9° of movement).

C4-5 and C6-7 inclusive and if they had never previously undergone cervical spinal surgery. As in previous studies, patients were assessed clinically, radiologically, and using an array of validated psychometric tests including the NDI, the SF-36, and a VAS relating to neck and arm pain. Adverse events were recorded and assessed according to World Health Organization recommendations. There was no significant difference in the number or distribution of adverse events between the two groups. At 12 months, the Prestige II disc maintained angular motion with a mean value of 5.9°. Both groups of patients showed improvement in NDI scores at 24 months compared with preoperative scores. Similarly, there were improvements in VAS scores and in general health status as assessed by the SF-36. The joint and fusion patients achieved similar scores. Based on these results, the use of the Prestige II disc is as safe and as efficacious as the standard Smith-Robinson fusion procedure [12]. The four-center study was the first to compare disc replacement technology with fusion in a prospective, randomized fashion.

Summary

Spine arthroplasty is a growing subspecialist area of spinal surgery. There are great opportunities for new materials, devices, and technology to emerge. TDR in the cervical spine offers the opportunity to preserve functional motion and maintain balance. It is postulated that arthroplasty may reduce adjacent-level disease more than traditional surgical treatment methods. The other advantages to this surgical option are immediate implant stability, no complications due to nonunion, and no need for graft harvesting.

The Bryan Cervical Disc is a metal-on-polymer implant with some elastic properties and a relatively mobile center of rotation. The Bristol Disc is a semi-constrained metal-on-metal prosthesis allowing AP translation motion of up to 2 mm. The ProDisc-C is a semiconstrained metal-polyethylene design allowing pure rotary motion that may stress the facet joints. Although there are no long-term data available yet, these three cervical prostheses appear promising in the nonfusion treatment of cervical degenerative disc disease.

References

[1] Pickett GE, Rouleau JP, Duggal N. Kinematic analysis of the cervical spine following implantation of an artificial cervical disc. Spine, in press.

[2] Lemaire J, Carrier H, Sari E, et al. The SB Charité III intervertebral disc prosthesis: radiological outcomes with a minimum 10-year follow-up. Presented at the annual meeting of the ISSLS. Porto, Portugal, June 2004.

[3] Goffin J, Casey A, Kehr P, et al. Preliminary clinical experience with the Bryan Cervical Disc Prosthesis. Neurosurgery 2002;51:840–5.

[4] Goffin J, Van Calenbergh V, van Loon J, et al. Intermediate follow-up after treatment of degenerative disc disease with the Bryan Cervical Disc Prosthesis: single-level and bi-level. Spine 2003;28:2673–8.

[5] Anderson PA, Sasso RC, Rouleau JP, et al. The Bryan Cervical Disc: wear properties and early clinical results. Spine J 2004;4:S303–9.

[6] Duggal N, Pickett GE, Mitsis DK, et al. Early clinical and biomechanical results following cervical arthroplasty. Neurosurg Focus 2004;17:62–8.

[7] Baron EM, Soliman AM, Gaughan JP, et al. Dysphagia, hoarseness, and unilateral true vocal fold motion impairment following anterior cervical diskectomy and fusion. Ann Otol Rhinol Laryngol 2003;112:921–6.

[8] Bazaz R, Lee MJ, Yoo JU. Incidence of dysphagia after anterior cervical spine surgery: a prospective study. Spine 2002;27:2453–8.

[9] Pickett GE, Sekhon LH, Sears W, et al. Early complications with cervical arthroplasty. J Neurosurg Spine, in press.

[10] Pickett GE, Mitsis DK, Sekhon LH, et al. Effects of a cervical disc prosthesis on segmental and cervical spine alignment. Neurosurg Focus 2004;17:30–5.

[11] Wigfield CC, Gill SS, Nelson RJ, et al. The new Frenchay artificial cervical joint: results from a two-year pilot study. Spine 2002;27:2446–52.

[12] Porchet F, Metcalf N. Clinical outcomes with the Prestige II Cervical Disc: preliminary results from a prospective randomised clinical trial. Neurosurg Focus 2004;17:36–43.

Posterior Dynamic Stabilization Systems: DYNESYS

Othmar Schwarzenbach, MD[a],*, Ulrich Berlemann, MD[a], Thomas M. Stoll, MD[b], Gilles Dubois, MD[c]

[a]dasRückenzentrum Thun, Bahnhofstrasse 3, 3600 Thun, Switzerland
[b]Bethesda Spital, 4020 Basel, Switzerland
[c]Nouvelle Clinique de l'Union, 31240 St. Jean, France

To reduce pain and disability, spinal surgery has always included three main components: decompression, stabilization, and correction of deformity. Various pathologic conditions necessitate combinations of these procedures, however, stabilization and fusion of spinal segments has become one of the most important principles in surgical treatment of spinal pathologies.

Initially, stabilization began with bony fusions and only later it was combined with some form of instrumentation. Following the early hardware augmentations by pioneers like Harrington for scoliosis surgery, Magerl with an external fixator for fracture treatment, Dick with an internal fixator, and Roy-Camille and Steffee with screw-plate systems, a wide array of fusion implants became available for every pathologic condition and every segment of the spine, for posterior as well as for anterior approaches [1–5]. These instrumentation techniques attempt a rigid stabilization to achieve solid fusion rather than the restoration of the function of segmental mobility. Fusion surgery can generate a considerable amount of morbidity and high rates of complications [6–9]. The elimination of mobility may overload adjacent segments, causing a high frequency of re-interventions [10–14]. Patient satisfaction after lumbar fusion has also been reported to be quite variable [15–17].

As a consequence, the search for alternative procedures was reinforced. A "dynamic stabilization" would ideally improve the movement and the load transfer of a spinal segment, without the intention of fusion. So far, various posterior dynamic stabilization systems have been described in the literature, such as interspinous distraction systems for stabilization after decompression procedures (Wallis, X STOP, DIAM), interspinous ligament devices (Loop system), or systems using ligaments across pedicle screws (Graf ligament) [18–22]. In particular during the last years, interspinous implants have gained some popularity. A recent prospective randomized multi-center study comparing the X STOP (ST. Francis Medical Technologies, Concord, California) with nonoperative treatment has shown favorable results for the surgical group after 1 year [19]. Senegas [23] published his initial results with the "Wallis system;" however, a randomized clinical trial was not yet available. Particularly in Europe, another flexible interspinous implant (DIAM, Medtronic, Sofamor Danek, Paris) is used for indications such as foraminal stenosis and disc protrusions, but up to now no prospective studies have been published.

The biomechanical background of stability concepts is based on the spinal motion segment. This was first defined by Junghanns [24] in 1968 and was later redefined on a precise biomechanical basis by White and Panjabi [25] in 1978, who introduced the term "functional spinal unit." The most obvious aspect of instability is excessive motion, but later nonphysiologic, abnormal motion was acknowledged and named "dysstability" [26].

This concept emphasized not only biomechanical considerations but also clinical signs and symptoms such as painful motion. With respect to the pathogenesis of spinal instability in degenerative spondy-

* Corresponding author.
E-mail address: o.schwarzenbach@dasrueckenzentrum.ch (O. Schwarzenbach).

losis, Kirkaldy-Willis and Farfan [27] presented in 1982 a convincing concept of three phases of degeneration: dysfunctional, unstable, and restabilization of the motion segment.

Considering these concepts of spinal instability and the history of instrumentation, the rationale for spinal stabilization can be defined as follows: diminishing pathologic motion, prevention of deformity, reduction of deformity, and compensation for iatrogenic destabilization. A dynamic stabilizing device ideally establishes painfree segmental motion and must withstand physiologic static and dynamic loads in any plane.

These concepts of instability causing low back pain are questioned by Mulholland and Sengupta [28]. They propose a concept where abnormal loading patterns due to disc disorganization occurring in degenerative disc disease are responsible for low back pain. Their "stone in the shoe" hypothesis—a degenerated disc is painful only at abnormal load transmission—is partially supported by modern results of fusion. If indeed instability was the main cause of back pain, one would have expected that spinal fusion would be more successful than it has been. Improvement in the instrumentation technique resulted in increase in successful fusion rate, but this has not been reflected by a corresponding increase in the rate of successful clinical outcome [29]. Mulholland and Sengupta [28] believe that dynamic stabilization systems work either because they restrict movement to a zone or range where normal or near normal loading may occur, or they prevent the spine adopting a position where abnormal loading may occur.

Philosophy and concept of DYNESYS

In 1994, Dubois and colleagues [30,31] for the first time implanted a pedicle screw-based system, with elastic, flexible connections, named DYNESYS (Dynamic Neutralization System for the Spine) (Fig. 1). DYNESYS intends to restore the biomechanics of the posterior annulus and facet joints and should thus allow for the reconstitution of the natural balance between the disc and posterior musculature. The system is designed to take into account the "three-phase concept of degeneration" of Kirkaldy-Willis, which combines a model of degeneration with different phases of instability. In the first unstable phase, the disc, with nuclear dehydration and annular weakening with protrusions and tears, loses its resistance to rotational and translational forces [32–35]. Subsequently, degeneration of the facet joints is

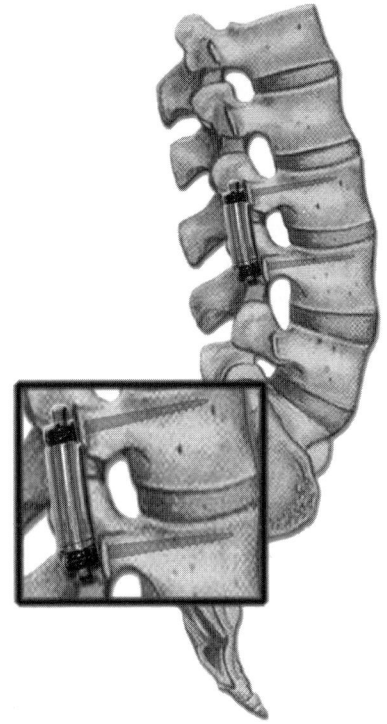

Fig. 1. Model of the Dynamic Neutralization System for the Spine. (*Courtesy of* Zimmer Spine, Minneapolis, Minnesota; with permission.)

induced with cartilage destruction and deformation to a more sagittal alignment. The loss of control over direction and restriction of motion contributes to further segmental instability. This is accompanied by the ligamentous laxity and muscular insufficiency. In the third and last phase, stability is eventually regained by disc collapse, osteochondrosis, spondylophytes, and locking of the facets while the segment is gradually ankylosing.

The first phase can be symptomatic with discogenic pain and even discal herniation. In the second phase patients may have pain in the disc, facets, and ligamentous structures. Additionally they may present with stenosis resulting from disc protrusion, facet joint growth, hypermobility, and deformity with ante- and retrolisthesis [36].

DYNESYS attempts to alter the late first phase and covers all mechanical aspects of the second phase. It reduces segmental motion to a physiologic level neutralizing bending, torsional, and shear forces. It should also unload the disc by reducing intradiscal pressure and the posterior annulus in particular. This appears important in reducing the strain on the annulus that may have become innervated in the course of degeneration, therefore being one cause of discogenic pain.

The DYNESYS system is composed of titanium alloy (Protasul-100) pedicle screws, polyethyleneterephthalate (Sulene-PET) cords, and polycarbonateurethane (Sulene-PCU) spacers. The screws anchor the DYNESYS system in the pedicle and in the vertebral body. The spacers fit between the pedicle screw heads. The stabilizing cords connect the pedicle screw heads via the hollow core of the spacer and hold the spacer in place (Fig. 2A, B). Their preload provides a uniform system rigidity. The stabilizing cords carry tensile forces (ie, during flexion movements), and spacers resist compressive forces. The inherent stability of the whole construct also resists bending and shear forces.

Several biomechanical in vitro experiments were conducted to study the efficacy of the system. One recently published study tested six lumbar cadaver spines, loading them with pure moments in the three motion planes [37]. The spines were tested intact, with a defect of the middle segment, stabilized with DYNESYS, and fixed with an internal fixator. For the bridged segment, the DYNESYS stabilized the spine and was more flexible than the internal fixator, particularly in extension where DYNESYS restored the range of motion to the intact condition. A second in vitro study found that increased spacer length increased the mobility in the segment [38]. In an animal model, motion increased after 6 months compared with the immediate postoperative state [39] and remained constant between 6 and 12 months.

A stabilization effect remained when the tests were performed after removal of DYNESYS. This indicates that the stiffness of the segment decreases within an initial period. In vivo measurements in DYNESYS patients, pre- and 6 months post-surgery, showed an increase in range of motion in one patient, no change in another, and a decrease in flexion and an increase in extension in a third. When the flexion-extension range of motion was measured using dynamic radiographs, the authors found that it was unchanged in 48% of the instrumented segments, decreased in 44%, and increased in 6% compared to the preoperative condition (O. Schwarzenbach, MD; T.M. Stoll, MD; G. Dubois, MD; unpublished data). This suggests that DYNESYS can either stabilize or maintain preoperative motion (preserve motion).

In addition to the biomechanical investigations, all individual components and interconnections were tested for their static as well as for their dynamic behavior to assess the safety of the system. Fatigue testing of the complete assembly was carried out for 10 million cycles, which is believed to represent a time in vivo of approximately 5 years. In an initial phase (one to two million cycles), the system showed stress relaxation and remained stable at a substantial load level afterwards. This also corresponds with the animal study by Cunningham [39], where in an initial phase the segmental stiffness decreased and then remained constant after 6 months.

The cord and spacer materials comply with the international standards of ISO 10993, and the pedicle screw exceeds those of ISO 5832-11. The nonmetallic parts were additionally tested in terms of biostability and degradation. PCU is known to have a high resistance to environmental stress cracking. An investigation of retrieved spacers (implantation time up to $5\frac{1}{2}$ years) has revealed no changes in chemical composition, molecular weight, and hardness when compared with a new, unimplanted spacer [40,41]. PET has not shown any degradation after $5\frac{1}{2}$ years in vivo [42].

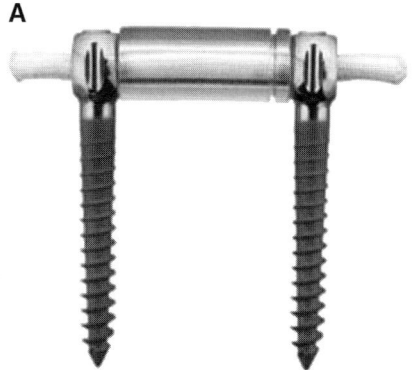
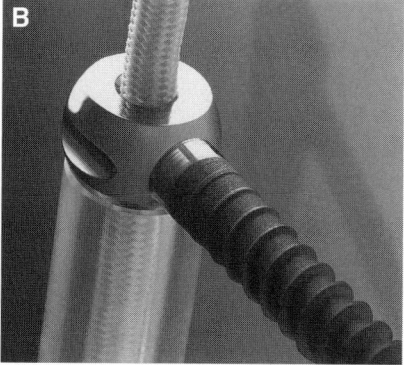

Fig. 2. (*A, B*) DYNESYS. (*Courtesy of* Zimmer Spine, Minneapolis, Minnesota; with permission.)

Indications

At the present time, posterior pedicular systems and distracting interspinous devices are used primarily for posterior dynamic stabilization. The indications for posterior dynamic stabilization devices are based on their design and biomechanical effects. Dynamic stabilization devices address instabilities of all kind: excessive or pathologic motion and gradually developing deformity, including iatrogenic instability. They address low back pain as well as neurogenic pain. Interspinous distraction devices are primarily indicated in degenerative disc disease and functional lumbar spinal stenosis, or to protect adjacent levels after spinal surgery implementing rigid spinal instrumentation [19,23,43].

The main goal of DYNESYS is to address dynamic instability in early stages of degeneration as defined by Kirkaldy-Willis [27]. As a result of the instability, the patient may experience several types of clinical symptoms. These include dynamic stenosis or stenosis with degenerative olisthesis as evidenced

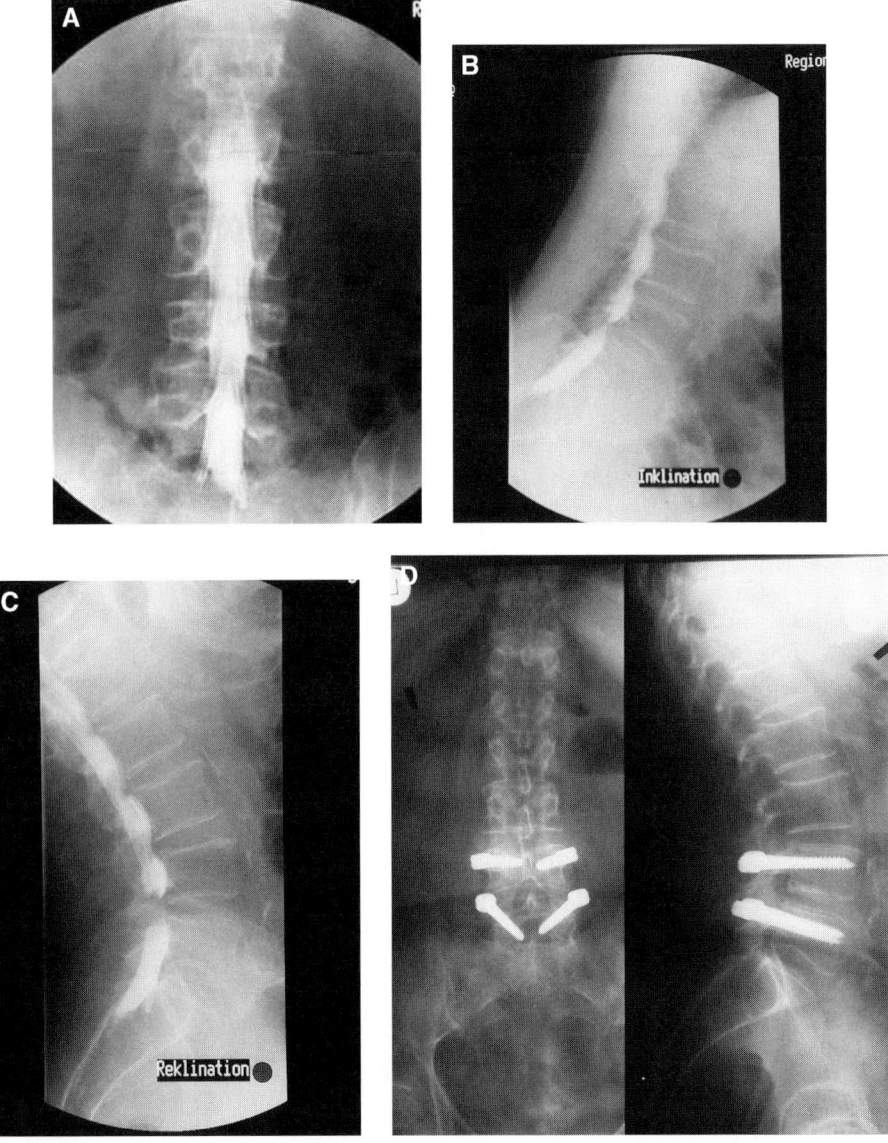

Fig. 3. Case 1: 63 year old female patient with dynamic stenosis. (*A–C*) Preoperative myelography. (*D*) Postoperative radiographs after implantation of DYNESYS.

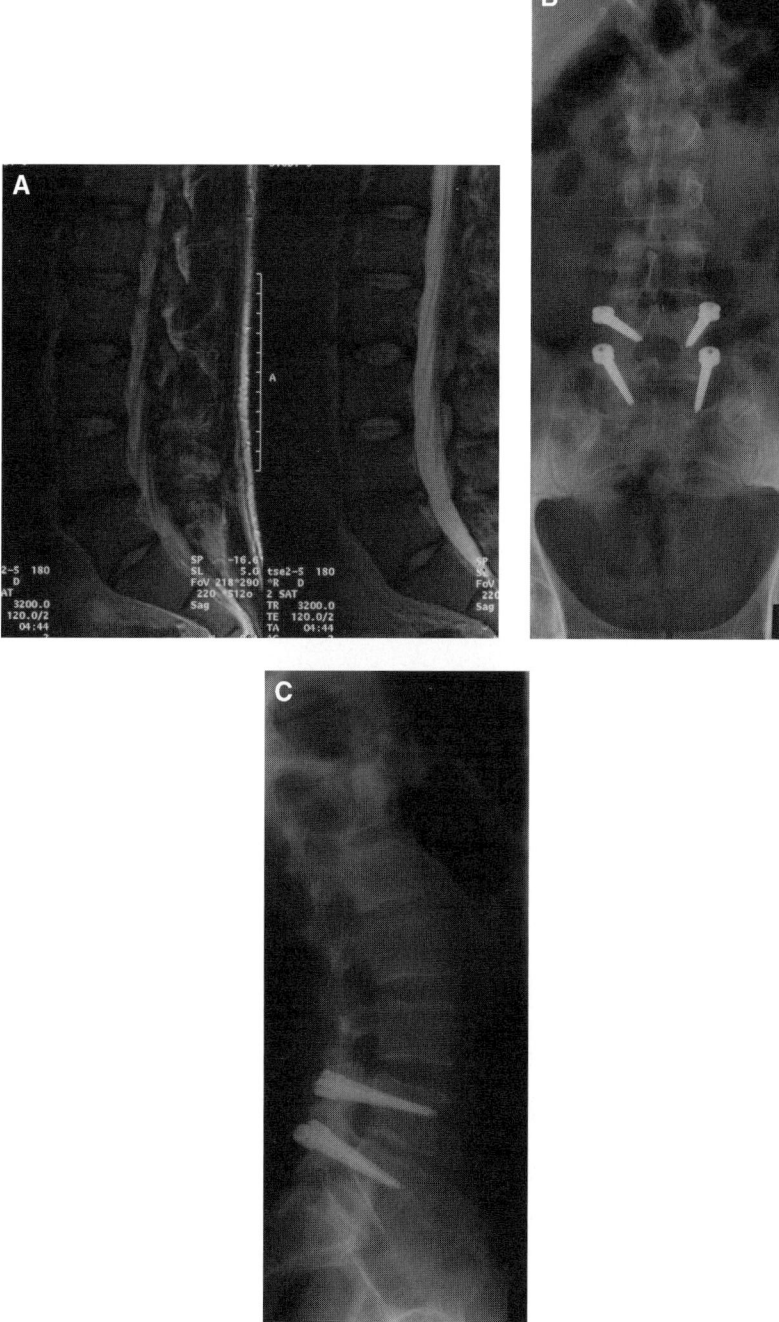

Fig. 4. Case 2: 36 year old male patient with discopathy and low back pain. Stabilization with DYNESYS after segment pathology was confirmed with a positive discography. (*A*) Preoperative MRI. (*B*) Anteroposterior radiograph 5 years postoperatively. (*C*) Lateral radiograph in reclination 5 years postoperatively.

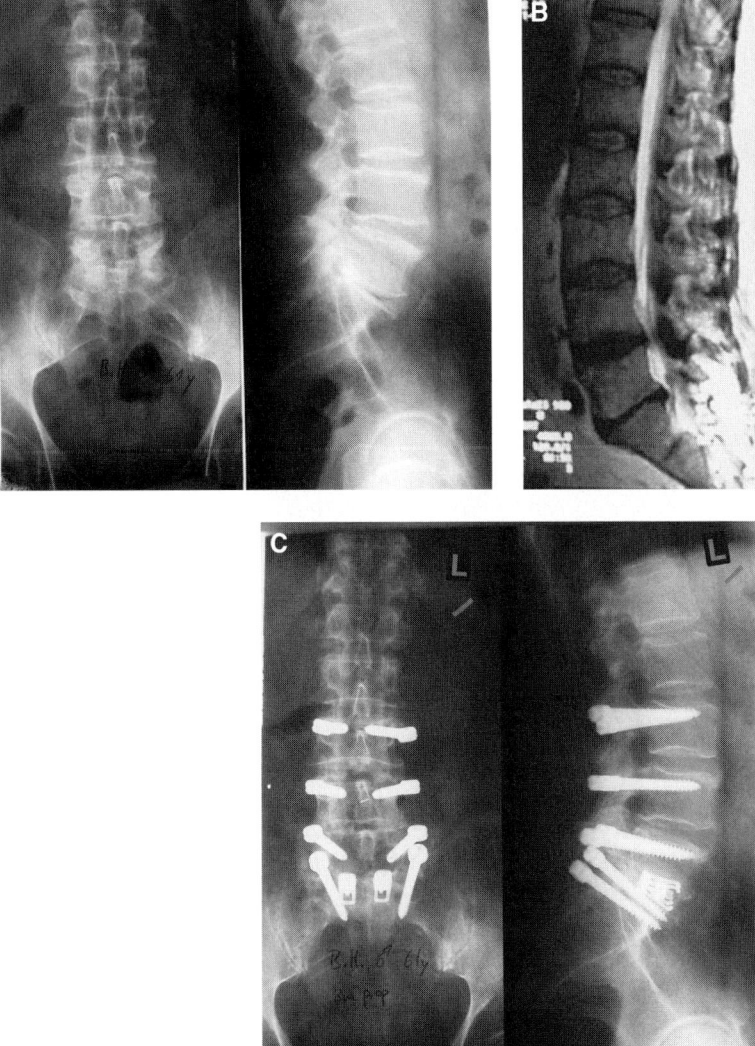

Fig. 5. Case 3: 61 year old male patient. Multisegmental degenerative disc disease with stenosis at L4/L5, severe disc degeneration at L5/S1. Underwent a PLIF L5/S1, DYNESYS L3-S1. (*A*) Preoperative radiographs. (*B*) Preoperative MRI. (*C*) Postoperative radiographs.

by neurogenic pain and/or low back pain (case presentation 1: Fig. 3A–D). Other indications for DYNESYS are mono- or multisegmental degenerative disc degeneration causing low back pain, iatrogenic instability following decompression and stenosis with early stages of gradually developing degenerative scoliosis (case presentation 2: Fig. 4A–C). In multilevel degenerative disc disease, DYNESYS may also be combined with a fusion procedure (e.g. PLIF), depending on the severity of segmental disc disruption (case presentation 3: Fig. 5A–C).

Clinical results with dynamic stabilization systems

Literature review reveals a lack of published data on most dynamic stabilization procedures. Senegas [23] has published a nonrandomized prospective study comparing 80 patients (two equal groups A and B) who underwent discectomy surgery for recurrence of herniated disc at L4/L5. One group (B) received a Wallis interspinous implant in addition to the decompression procedure. The mean follow-up was 3 years and 4 months. The percentage of improvement in low back pain over the preoperative visual analog scale (VAS) score at follow-up was 52% in group A (discectomy alone) and 74% in group B (discectomy and Wallis implant). Nerve root pain was improved by 87% (A) and 92% (B). Oswestry Disability Index (ODI) changed in group A from 54.7% to 22% and in group B from 58.2% to 16.4%. Overall five patients underwent reoperations (three fusion, two decompressions) during the follow-up time. Senegas [23] concludes that nonrigid fixation appears to be a useful technique in the management of initial forms of degenerative intervertebral lumbar disc disease.

Zucherman et al [19] recently published preliminary results from a prospective, randomized trial of the X STOP conducted at nine centers in the United States. Two hundred patients were enrolled in the study and 191 were treated; 100 received the X STOP and 91 received nonoperative therapy (NON OP) as a control. The Zurich Claudication Questionnaire (ZCQ) was the primary outcomes measurement. Validated for lumbar spinal stenosis patients, the ZCQ measures physical function, symptom severity, and patient satisfaction. Patients completed the ZCQ on enrollment and at follow-up periods of 6 weeks, 6 months, and 1 year. Using the ZCQ criteria, at 6 weeks the success rate was 52% for X STOP patients and 10% for NON OP patients. At 6 months, the success rates were 52% and 9%, respectively, and at 1 year, 59% and 12%. The results of this prospective study indicate that the X STOP offers a significant improvement over nonoperative therapies at 1 year with a success rate comparable to published reports for decompressive laminectomy, but with considerably lower morbidity. Lee et al [44] have also published good results for X-STOP to treat lumbar spinal stenosis in a small patient group with a short follow-up.

Stoll et al [45] presented their first results with DYNESYS in 2002. The prospective, multicenter study evaluated the safety and efficacy of DYNESYS to treat lumbar instability conditions, evaluating pre- and postoperative pain, function, and radiologic data on a consecutive series of 83 patients. Unstable segmental conditions were mainly combined with spinal stenosis (60.2%) and with degenerative discopathy (24.1%), in some cases with disc herniation (8.4%), and with revision surgery (6.0%). Thirty-nine patients additionally had degenerative spondylolisthesis and 30 patients had previous lumbar surgery. In 56 patients instrumentation was combined with direct decompression. The mean age at operation was 58.2 (26.8 to 85.3) years, the mean follow-up time was 38.1 months (11.2 to 79.1). Nine complications were unrelated to the implant and one due to a screw malplacement. Four of them needed an early surgical reintervention. Additional lumbar surgery in the follow-up period included implant removal and conversion into spinal fusion with rigid instrumentation for persisting pain in three cases, laminectomy of an index segment in one case, and screw removal due to loosening in one case. In seven patients, adjacent segment degeneration necessitated further surgery. Mean pain and function scores improved significantly from baseline to follow-up: back pain scale from 7.4 to 3.1, leg pain scale 6.9 to 2.4, Oswestry Disability Index 55.4% to 22.9%. The authors [45] conclude that these study results are comparable with those obtained by conventional procedures; however, mobile stabilization is less invasive than fusion. Long-term screw fixation depends on correct screw dimension and proper screw positioning. The natural course of polysegmental disease in some cases necessitates further surgery as the disease progresses. Dynamic neutralization proved to be a safe and effective alternative in the treatment of unstable lumbar conditions.

Positive results about the application of DYNESYS in patients with degenerative disc disease have been published by Putzier et al [46] in 2004. They concluded that DYNESYS is able to compensate initial morphologic changes and prevent progression of segment degeneration. They conclude that DYNESYS does not appear to be indicated for treating marked deformities or if osseous decompression needs to be performed.

Cakir et al [47] published a retrospective study where they analyzed the outcome of patients with degenerative lumbar instability with spinal stenosis who underwent decompression surgery with dorsoventral fusion or decompression surgery with posterior dynamic stabilization. In a small group of patients (n = 20), the DYNESYS group showed a slightly better outcome and shorter operation time and hospital stay. Cakir et al [47] conclude that dynamic stabilization appears to be a promising alternative to fusion in patients with degenerative instability with spinal stenosis.

Currently, the authors' series on patients with degenerative disc disease (DDD) and stenosis treated with DYNESYS is being summarized and will be published soon (T.M. Stoll, MD; O. Schwarzenbach,

MD; G. Dubois, MD; unpublished data). DYNESYS is not indicated as a primary stabilization method in lytic (isthmic) spondylolisthesis and severe degenerative scoliotic or kyphotic deformation.

Currently, 20 U.S. sites are participating in a Food and Drug Administration (FDA) Investigational Device Exemption (IDE) multicenter prospective randomized clinical trial evaluating the safety and effectiveness of DYNESYS. More than 400 DYNESYS patients have been enrolled so far. The enrollment should be complete by spring 2005.

Summary

Posterior dynamic stabilization systems have to neutralize injurious forces and restore painless function of the spine segments and protect the adjacent segments. Dynamic stabilization systems will play an important role in the treatment of degenerative lumbar spine. Because degenerative disc disease has many clinical manifestations, pedicular screw systems and interspinous implants have their indications. The cause of low back pain in degenerative disc disease is still a mystery. Many theories try to explain the connections between low back pain and the degenerative cascade of the motion segment. Because the theoretical background is incomplete, the actual designs of all these novel implants can not be perfect. A dynamic stabilization device has to provide stability throughout its lifetime unless it activates or allows reparative processes with a reversal of the degenerative changes. Anchorage to the bone is crucial, at least for pedicular systems. This is a great demand on spinal implants and assumes rest and motion going together. Our experience with DYNESYS has shown that this method has limitations in elderly patients with osteoporotic bone or in patients with a severe segmental macro-instability combined with degenerative olisthesis and advanced disc degeneration. Such cases have an increased risk of failure. Only future randomized evaluations will be able to address the potential reduction of accelerated adjacent segment degeneration.

The few posterior dynamic stabilization systems that have had clinical applications so far have produced clinical outcomes comparable with fusion. No severe adverse events caused by these implants have been reported. Long-term follow-up data and controlled prospective randomized studies are not available for most of the cited implants but are essential to prove the safety, efficacy, appropriateness and economic viability of these methods.

References

[1] Harrington PR, Dickson JH. Spinal instrumentation in the treatment of severe progressive spondylolisthesis. Clin Orthop 1976;117:157–63.

[2] Magerl F. Stabilization of the lower thoracic and lumbar spine with external skeletal fixation. Clin Orthop 1984;189:125–41.

[3] Dick W, Kluger P, Magerl F, et al. A new device for internal fixation of thoracolumbar and lumbar spine fractures: the "fixateur interne." Paraplegia 1985;23(4):225–32.

[4] Roy-Camille R, Saillant G, Berteaux D, et al. [Vertebral osteosynthesis using metal plates. Its different uses]. Chirurgie 1979;105(7):597–603 [in French].

[5] Steffee AD, Biscup RS, Sitkowski DJ. Segmental spine plates with pedicular fixation. A new internal fixation device for disorders of the lumbar and thoracolumbar spine. Clin Orthop 1986;203:45–53.

[6] Christensen FB. Lumbar spinal fusion: outcome in relation to surgical methods, choice of implant and postoperative rehabilitation. Acta Orthop Scand Suppl 2004;74(313):1–43.

[7] Fritzell P, Hagg O, Nordwall A, Swedish Lumbar Spine Study Group. Complications in lumbar fusion surgery for chronic low back pain: comparison of three surgical techniques used in a prospective randomized study. A report from the Swedish Lumbar Spine Study Group. Eur Spine J 2003;26(5 Suppl):S545–8.

[8] Rompe JD, Eysel P, Zollner J, et al. Degenerative lumbar spinal stenosis. Long-term results after undercutting decompression compared with decompressive laminectomy alone or with instrumented fusion. Neurosurg Rev 1999;22(2–3):102–6.

[9] Whitecloud 3rd TS, Davis JM, Olive PM. Operative treatment of the degenerated segment adjacent to a lumbar fusion. Spine 1994;19(5):531–6.

[10] Aota Y, Kumano K, Hirabayashi S. Postfusion instability at the adjacent segments after rigid pedicle screw fixation for degenerative lumbar spinal disorders. J Spinal Disord 1995;8(6):464–73.

[11] Rahm MD, Hall BB. Adjacent-segment degeneration after lumbar fusion with instrumentation: a retrospective study. J Spinal Disord 1996;9(6):392–400.

[12] Schlegel JD, Smith JA, Schleusener RL. Lumbar motion segment pathology adjacent to thoracolumbar, lumbar, and lumbosacral fusions. Spine 1996;21(8):970–81.

[13] Schulitz KP, Wiesner L, Wittenberg RH, Hille E. [The mobile segment above fusion]. Z Orthop Ihre Grenzgeb 1996;134(2):171–6 [in German].

[14] Lehmann TR, Spratt KF, Tozzi JE, et al. Long-term follow-up of lower lumbar fusion patients. Spine 1987;12(2):97–104.

[15] Buttermann GR, Garvey TA, Hunt AF, et al. Lumbar fusion results related to diagnosis. Spine 1998;23(1):116–27.

[16] Turner JA, Ersek M, Herron L, et al. Patient

outcomes after lumbar spinal fusions. JAMA 1992; 268(7):907–11.
[17] Thomsen K, Christensen FB, Eiskjaer SP, et al. 1997 Volvo Award winner in clinical studies. The effect of pedicle screw instrumentation on functional outcome and fusion rates in posterolateral lumbar spinal fusion: a prospective randomized clinical study. Spine 1997; 22(24):2813–22.
[18] Senegas J, Etchevers JP, Vital JM, et al. [Recalibration of the lumbar canal, an alternative to laminectomy in the treatment of lumbar canal stenosis]. Rev Chir Orthop Reparatrice Appar Mot 1988;74(1):15–22 [in French].
[19] Zucherman JF, Hsu KY, Hartjen CA, et al. A prospective randomized multi-center study for the treatment of lumbar spinal stenosis with the X STOP interspinous implant: 1-year results. Eur Spine J 2004; 13(1):22–31.
[20] Caserta S, La Maida GA, Misaggi B, et al. Elastic stabilization alone or combined with rigid fusion in spinal surgery: a biomechanical study and clinical experience based on 82 cases. Eur Spine J 2002; 11(Suppl 2):S192–7.
[21] Garner MD, Wolfe SJ, Kuslich SD. Development and preclinical testing of a new tension-band device for the spine: the Loop system. Eur Spine J 2002;11(Suppl 2): S186–91.
[22] Graf H. Lumbar instability. Surgical treatment without fusion. Rachis 1992;412:123–37.
[23] Senegas J. Mechanical supplementation by non-rigid fixation in degenerative intervertebral lumbar segments: the Wallis system. Eur Spine J 2002;11(Suppl 2): S164–9.
[24] Junghanns H. Die gesunde und die kranke Wirbelsäule in Röntgenbild und Klinik. Stuttgart: Thieme; 1968.
[25] White 3rd AA, Panjabi MM. The basic kinematics of the human spine. A review of past and current knowledge. Spine 1978;3(1):12–20.
[26] Olerud S, Sjöström L, Karlström G, Hamberg M. Spontaneous effect of increased stability of the lower lumbar spine in cases of severe chronic back pain. The answer of external transpeduncular fixation test. Clin Orthop 1986;203:67–74.
[27] Kirkaldy-Willis WH, Farfan HF. Instability of the lumbar spine. Clin Orthop 1982;165:110–23.
[28] Mulholland RC, Sengupta DK. Rationale, principles and experimental evaluation of the concept of soft stabilization. Eur Spine J 2002;11(Suppl 2): S198–205.
[29] Boos N, Webb JK. Pedicle screw fixation in spinal disorders: a European view. Eur Spine J 1997;6(1): 2–18.
[30] Dubois G, De Germay B, Schaerer NS, Fennema P. Dynamic neutralization: a new concept for restabilization of the spine. In: Szpalski M, Gunzburg R, Pope MH, editors. Lumbar segmental instability. Philadelphia: Lippincott Williams & Wilkins; 1999. p. 233–40.
[31] Freudiger S, Dubois G, Lorrain M. Dynamic neutralization of the lumbar spine confirmed on a new lumbar spine simulator in vitro. Arch Orthop Trauma Surg 1999;119:127–32.
[32] Niosi CA, Oxland TR. Degenerative mechanics of the lumbar spine. Spine 2004;4(6 Suppl):202S–8S.
[33] Fujiwara A, Lim TH, An HS, et al. The relationship between disc degeneration and facet joint osteoarthritis on the segmental flexibility of the lumbar spine. Spine 2000;25:3036–44.
[34] Fujiwara A, Tamai K, An HS, et al. The relationship between disc degeneration, facet joint osteoarthritis, and stability of the degenerative lumbar spine. J Spinal Disord 2000;13:444–50.
[35] Farfan HF, Huberdeau RM, Dubow HI. Lumbar intervertebral disc degeneration: the influence of geometrical features on the pattern of disc degeneration—a post mortem study. J Bone Joint Surg Am 1972; 54(3):492–519.
[36] Frymoyer JW, Selby DK. Segmental instability. Rationale for treatment. Spine 1985;10(3):280–6.
[37] Schmoelz W, Huber JF, Nydegger T, et al. Dynamic stabilization of the lumbar spine and its effects on adjacent segments: an in vitro experiment. J Spinal Disord Tech 2003;16(4):418–23.
[38] Niosi C, Zhu Q, Wilson D, et al. Does spacer length of dynamic posterior stabilization system have an effect on kinematic behaviour? SAS annual meeting, May 4–7, 2004, Vienna, Austria.
[39] Cunningham B, Dmitriev A, Hu N, et al. Pre-clinical evaluation of a dynamic posterior spinal stabilization system (Dynesys™): A non-human primate model. ISSLS annual meeting, May 30–June 5, 2004, Porto, Portugal.
[40] Trommsdorff U, Zurbrügg D, Schneider W. In-vivo degradation behavior of polycarbonate-urethane in a spinal implant system. Transactions of the 29th Annual Meeting of the Society of Biomaterials. Reno, Nevada, May 3, 2003.
[41] Trommsdorff U, Zurbrügg D, Stoll TM. In-vivo stability of polycarbonate-urethane with and without contact to an abscess. Transactions of the 7th World Biomaterials Congress. Sydney, Australia, May 17–21, 2004.
[42] Trommsdorff U, Zurbrügg D, Schneider W. Biostability of poly(ethylene-terephthalate) cords used in a spinal implant system. Transactions of the 7th World Biomaterials Congress. Sydney, Australia, May 17–21, 2004.
[43] Kaech DL, Fernandez C, Lombardi-Weber D. The interspinous 'U': a new restabilization device for the lumbar spine. In: Kaech DL, Jinkins JR, editors. Spinal restabilization procedures. Diagnostic and therapeutic aspects of intervertebral fusion cages, artificial discs and mobile implants. Amsterdam: Elsevier Science B.V.; 2002. p. 355–62.
[44] Lee J, Hida K, Seki T, et al. An interspinous process distractor (X STOP) for lumbar spinal stenosis in elderly patients: preliminary experiences in 10 consecutive cases. J Spinal Disord Tech 2004;17(1):72–7.

[45] Stoll TM, Dubois G, Schwarzenbach O. The dynamic neutralization system for the spine: a multi-center study of a novel non-fusion system. Eur Spine J 2002;11(Suppl 2):S170–8.

[46] Putzier M, Schneider SV, Funk J, Perka C. [Application of a dynamic pedicle screw system (DYNESYS) for lumbar segmental degenerations—comparison of clinical and radiological results for different indications]. Z Orthop Ihre Grenzgeb 2004;142(2):166–73 [in German].

[47] Cakir B, Ulmar B, Koepp H, et al. Posterior dynamic stabilization as an alternative for instrumented fusion in the treatment of degenerative lumbar instability with spinal stenosis. Z Orthop 2003;141:418–24.

Rationale, Biomechanics, and Surgical Indications for Graf Ligamentoplasty

Masahiro Kanayama, MD*, Tomoyuki Hashimoto, MD, Keiichi Shigenobu, MD

Department of Orthopaedic Surgery, Hakodate Central General Hospital, Hon-cho 33-2, Hakodate, Hokkaido 040-8585, Japan

In the past, posterolateral fusion has been widely used to treat degenerative lumbar disorders [1–4]; however, spinal fusion increases mechanical stress at the segments adjacent to the fusion level [5,6]. Clinically, the results of several long-term follow-up studies have suggested that spinal fusion might cause deterioration of the adjacent segment [7–9]. Limitations and problems with spinal fusion have led some investigators to explore nonfusion technologies [10–12].

Graf artificial ligament stabilization (SEM Co., Mountrouge, France) can ideally be used to stabilize the unstable segment without rigid spinal fusion. The Graf system is composed of 5- to 7-mm titanium pedicle screws and looped 8-mm braided polyester bands (Fig. 1). Under applied compressive force between the pedicle screws, the bands are connected to the screws to stabilize the operative segment in lordosis. The concepts of Graf artificial ligament stabilization include (1) immobilization in lordosis, providing stability through coaptation of the facet joints; (2) alteration of annular and end plate load bearing; (3) posterior annular compression, resulting in closure of annular tears; (4) splinting of the motion segment, allowing healing of damaged tissue; and (5) band relaxation over the first 4 to 6 months, allowing some return to movement [12]. In addition, Gardner [13] suggested the following advantages of Graf ligamentoplasty over spinal arthrodesis: (1) it is less invasive and more physiologically sound so it encourages better neuromuscular recovery and reduces stress on adjacent discs; (2) it has a shorter operation time and less blood loss compared with instrumented spinal fusion; (3) there is no or minimal external support required postoperatively; and (4) there is no risk of pseudarthrosis or donor-site pain because no bone grafting procedures are required.

Biomechanics

Several biomechanical investigations were conducted regarding the effect of Graf ligament stabilization [14–16]. Strauss et al [14] investigated the biomechanical influences of the Graf fixation system on spinal motion segments using a human cadaveric lumbar spine model. The data showed that the Graf system significantly reduced angular motion in flexion–extension but had little effect on the translation of the vertebral body in any direction. This finding suggested that Graf ligament stabilization had the potential to treat "flexion instability" but had limited ability to reduce or prevent spondylolisthesis.

Wild et al [15] reported in an ex vivo biomechanical study that rotational instabilities cannot satisfactorily be stabilized by Graf ligamentoplasty. This study showed that the procedure also had limitations in restoration of rotational stability and in reducing scoliotic or rotational deformity.

* Corresponding author.
E-mail address: mkanayama@aol.com (M. Kanayama).

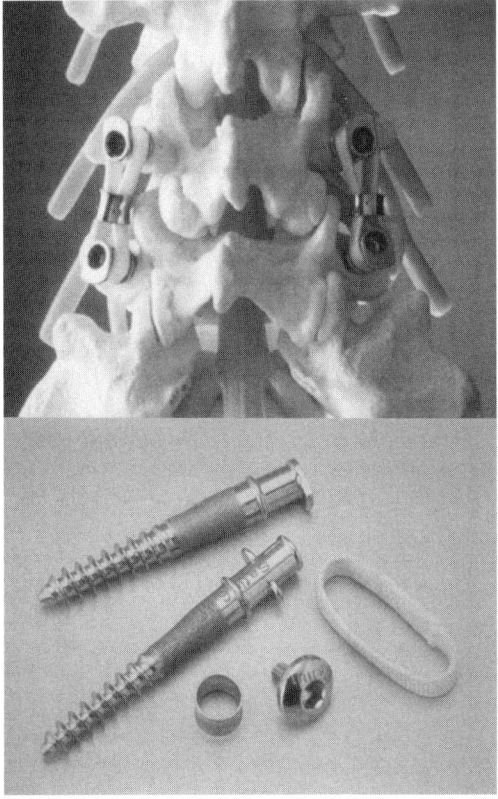

Fig. 1. Graf artificial ligament instrumentation. (*Courtesy of* Showaika Kogyo, Co., Japan; with permission.)

Hasegawa et al [16] investigated the role of facet joints on the stability provided by the Graf system. Using a porcine spine model, these investigators demonstrated that unilateral facetectomy significantly reduced the rotational stability of Graf ligamentoplasty. This procedure provided stability through coaptation of the bilateral facet joints; facet joints and the intervertebral disc are key structures for successful ligamentoplasty.

Surgical indications

Graf ligamentoplasty is not a procedure that can completely replace spinal arthrodesis. Appropriate surgical indication and patient selection are imperative to obtain successful clinical outcomes. The authors' surgical indication for Graf ligamentoplasty is degenerative lumbar disorders with less than 25% of vertebral slippage, minimal disc space narrowing, and coronal facet articulation (Fig. 2). High-grade spondylolisthesis cannot be reduced and stabilized by the Graf system alone; the indication for this procedure should be limited to grade I or less olisthesis. The intervertebral disc is a key structure to support the anterior column when applying compressive force to the pedicle screws; the disc space should be preserved to avoid iatrogenic neuroforaminal stenosis. The facet joint is another key structure. Because this procedure provides stability through coaptation of the bilateral facet joints, tropism of the facet articulation should be coronal.

Contraindications are listed in Box 1. Isthmic spondylolisthesis often requires bilateral facetectomies and foraminotomies and, therefore, facet joints cannot serve as a fulcrum. Retrolisthesis is a contraindication for Graf ligamentoplasty because ligamentoplasty cannot restore extension stability and retrolisthesis may increase when applying compressive force between the pedicle screws. Laterolisthesis and scoliosis are not indicated for ligamentoplasty. Vertebral slippage and rotational instability cannot be reduced by this procedure. Patients with disc space narrowing or neuroforaminal stenosis are not candidates for this procedure. In such cases, neuroforaminal stenosis is worsened by applied compressive force. Rigid kyphotic deformity is also difficult to correct with the Graf system and requires extensive reconstruction by interbody fusion or osteotomy. Sagittal facet tropism is not appropriate for Graf ligamentoplasty because such facet joints cannot function as a mechanical restraint to anterolisthesis, which may progress. Obese patients and manual laborers place excessive biomechanical demands on the Graf ligamentoplasty and are at risk for mechanical failure of the device.

In the authors' series [17,18], all patients had sciatic symptoms or neurogenic claudication due to spinal stenosis or herniated disc. The authors did not perform this procedure for the patients who had only low back pain and degenerative disc disease. Because low back pain and sciatic symptoms were improved in this series, however, Graf ligamentoplasty may have a potential to alleviate low back pain in patients with degenerative disc disease.

Modic change and dark disc on MRI are significant factors in patient selection. Preserved disc height is the most important parameter regarding intervertebral disc status. In the authors' series [18], the percentage of posterior disc height to the lower vertebral height (percent posterior disc height) ranged from 17% to 40% and averaged to 28% preoperatively.

Failed back surgeries or recurrent disc herniation are not contraindications to Graf ligamentoplasty;

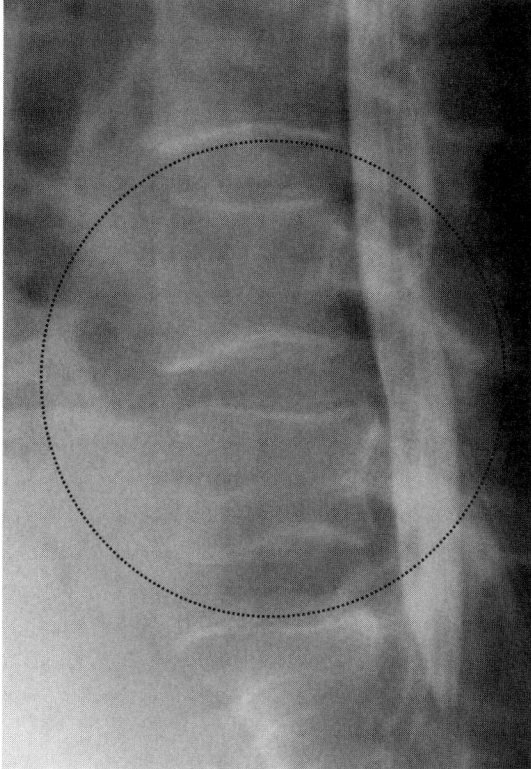 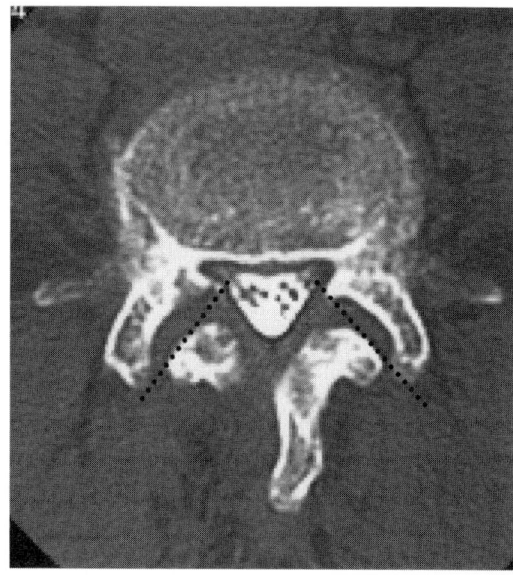

Fig. 2. Surgical indications for Graf ligamentoplasty include symptomatic degenerative lumbar disorder with less than 25% of vertebral slip (*left*), minimal disc space narrowing (*left*), and coronal facet articulation (*right*).

however, as mentioned previously, facet joints must be preserved bilaterally during the decompression procedure. If complete facetectomy is required even unilaterally, the authors recommend instrumented fusion instead of Graf ligamentoplasty.

Box 1. Contraindication for Graf ligamentoplasty

Isthmic spondylolisthesis
Retro listhesis
Lateral slip of vertebra
Scoliosis deformity
Disc space narrowing (with foraminal stenosis)
Rigid kyphotic deformity
Sagittal facet tropism
Obesity
Heavy worker

Clinical results

Several clinical studies have reported that Graf artificial ligament stabilization provides significant improvement of low back pain symptoms [12,17,19,20]. In the initial report by Graf [12], 80% of the 120 patients followed for 6 to 24 months were satisfied with the results of this procedure. Although there was enthusiasm over the early clinical results obtained with Graf artificial ligament stabilization, the associated mid- to long-term results remain controversial [21]. Hadlow et al [21] investigated the clinical results of 83 patients who underwent Graf ligamentoplasty or posterolateral lumbar fusion and reported that ligamentoplasty was associated with a worse outcome and a significantly higher revision rate than posterolateral fusion with pedicle screw instrumentation. Variability of published results may largely depend on differences in indications and patient selection.

The authors have performed Graf ligamentoplasty under the aforementioned surgical indications since

1994. Midterm clinical results were reported in two peer-reviewed publications. Hashimoto et al [17] investigated radiographic and clinical outcomes of Graf ligamentoplasty in 59 patients with lumbar flexion instability; they concluded that this procedure could stabilize the unstable segment without rigid spinal arthrodesis and was a successful alternative to spinal arthrodesis in a patient population with less than 10° of flexion instability. Kanayama et al [18] also reviewed 64 patients with degenerative spondylolisthesis treated by Graf ligamentoplasty. At minimum 2-year follow-up, Graf ligament stabilization maintained lordosis and preserved segmental motion in most cases. Although vertebral slippage was not improved by this procedure, progressive postoperative disc space narrowing did not occur. Revision surgery was required at the ligamentoplasty level in only 1.6% of patients. Although no attempt was made to achieve fusion, facet fusion occurred spontaneously in 18.8% of patients at average 59.5 months after surgery.

Although controversy over the mid- to long-term clinical outcomes still exists, because Graf ligamentoplasty is a "motion-preserving" technology, it has the potential to reduce the risk of adjacent-segment morbidity compared with arthrodesis. Kanayama et al [22] investigated the prevalence of adjacent-segment disease after Graf ligamentoplasty versus instrumented posterolateral lumbar fusion. Data were obtained in 45 patients who underwent L4-5 Graf ligamentoplasty (18 patients) or instrumented posterolateral lumbar fusion (27 patients). Radiographic evidence of adjacent-disc deterioration was observed more frequently in patients with fusion than with ligamentoplasty (Fig. 3). At a minimum 5-year follow-up, the prevalence of adjacent-segment disease requiring reoperation was 5.6% in Graf ligamentoplasty and 18.5% in posterolateral lumbar fusion. In this study, Graf ligamentoplasty seemed to reduce the risk of adjacent-segment deterioration.

Summary

Graf ligamentoplasty stabilizes the unstable segment through coaptation of bilateral facet joints. Intervertebral disc height should be preserved to avoid postoperative neuroforaminal stenosis. Biomechanically and clinically, this procedure has the potential to treat flexion instability but cannot correct vertebral slippage or scoliotic deformity.

Surgical indication or patient selection is the key to successful ligamentoplasty. The surgical indication is degenerative lumbar disorder with less than 25% of vertebral slip, minimal disc space narrowing, and coronal facet tropism. In the long-term, Graf ligamentoplasty may reduce the risk of adjacent-segment deterioration compared with spinal fusion.

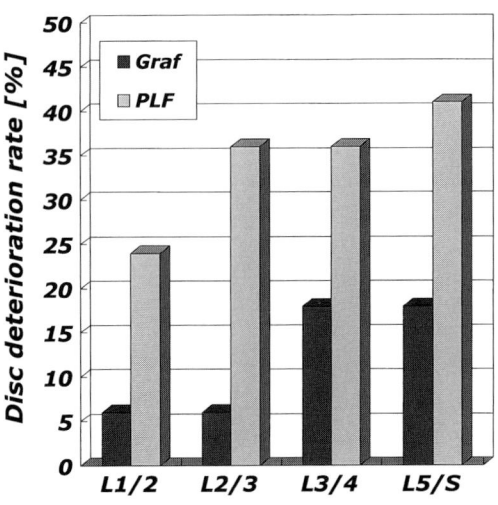

Fig. 3. Radiographic assessment of adjacent-disc deterioration after Graf ligamentoplasty versus instrumented posterolateral fusion (PLF). A higher rate of adjacent-disc deterioration was found in the PLF group compared with the Graf group.

References

[1] Bridwell KH, Sedgewick TA, O'Brien MF, et al. The role of fusion and instrumentation in the treatment of degenerative spondylolisthesis with spinal stenosis. J Spinal Disord 1993;6:461–72.
[2] Kaneda K, Kazama H, Satoh S, et al. Follow up study of medial facetectomies and posterolateral fusion with instrumentation in unstable degenerative spondylolisthesis. Clin Orthop 1986;203:159–67.
[3] West III JL, Bradford DS, Ogilvie JW. Results of spinal arthrodesis with pedicle screw-plate fixation. J Bone Joint Surg Am 1991;73:1179–84.
[4] Zdeblick TA. A prospective, randomized study of lumbar fusion: preliminary results. Spine 1993;18:983–91.
[5] Cunningham BW, Kotani Y, McNulty PS, et al. The effect of spinal destabilization and instrumentation on lumbar intradiscal pressure: an in vitro biomechanical analysis. Spine 1997;22:2655–63.
[6] Lee CK, Langrana NA. Lumbosacral spinal fusion: a biomechanical study. Spine 1984;9:574–81.
[7] Lee CK. Accelerated degeneration of the segment adjacent to a lumbar fusion. Spine 1988;13:375–7.
[8] Lehmann TR, Spratt KF, Tozzi JE, et al. Long-term follow-up of lower lumbar fusion patients. Spine 1987;12:97–104.

[9] Leong JC, Chun SY, Grange WJ, et al. Long-term results of lumbar intervertebral disc prolapse. Spine 1983;8:793–9.

[10] Ray CD. The PDN prosthetic disc-nucleus device. Eur Spine J 2002;11:S137–42.

[11] Cinotti G, David T, Postacchini F. Results of disc prosthesis after a minimum follow-up period of 2 years. Spine 1996;21:995–1000.

[12] Graf H. Lumbar instability. Surgical treatment without fusion. Rachis 1992;412:123–37.

[13] Gardner ADH. An alternative concept in the surgical management of lumbar degenerative disc disease-flexible stabilization. In: Margulies JY, editor. Lumbosacral and spinopelvic fixation. Philadelphia: Lippincot-Raven; 1992. p. 889–905.

[14] Strauss PJ, Novotny JE, Wilder DG, et al. Multidirectional stability of the Graf system. Spine 1994;19:965–72.

[15] Wild A, Jaeger M, Bushe C, et al. Biomechanical analysis of Graf's dynamic spine stabilisation system ex vivo. Biomed Tech (Berl) 2001;46:290–4.

[16] Hasegawa K, Takano K, Endo N, et al. [A biomechanical study on the stabilizing effect of Graf ligamentoplasty in a graded destabilization model of porcine lumbar spine]. Rinsho Seikei Geka 2004;39:133–40 [in Japanese].

[17] Gardner A, Pande KC. Graf ligamentoplasty: a 7-year follow-up. Eur Spine J 2002;11:S157–63.

[18] Hashimoto T, Oha F, Shigenobu K, et al. Mid-term clinical results of Graf stabilization for lumbar degenerative pathologies: a minimum 2-year follow-up. Spine J 2001;1:283–9.

[19] Moon MS, Moon YW, Moon JL, et al. Treatment of flexion instability of lumbar spine with Graf band. J Musculoskeletal Res 1999;3:49–63.

[20] Hadlow SV, Fagan AB, Hillier TM, et al. The Graf ligamentoplasty procedure. Comparison with posterolateral fusion in the management of low back pain. Spine 1998;23:1172–9.

[21] Kanayama M, Hashimoto T, Shigenobu K, et al. Non-fusion surgery for degenerative spondylolisthesis using artificial ligament stabilization: surgical indication and clinical results. Spine 2005;30:588–92.

[22] Kanayama M, Hashimoto T, Shigenobu K, et al. Adjacent-segment morbidity after Graf ligamentoplasty compared with posterolateral lumbar fusion. J Neurosurg 2001;95(Suppl 1):5–10.

Hybrid Constructs

Rudolf Bertagnoli, MD[a],*, Patrick Tropiano, MD, PhD[b], Jack Zigler, MD[c], Armin Karg, MSc[d], Sandra Voigt, MSc[d]

[a]*Spine Center, St.-Elisabeth-Klinikum, St.-Elisabeth-Str. 23, 94315 Straubing, Germany*
[b]*Aix-Marseille University, Hôpital Nord, Chemin des Bourrelly, 13915 Marseille cedex 20, France*
[c]*Texas Back Institute, 6300 West Parker Road, Plano, TX 75093-7916, USA*
[d]*Spine Center Straubing, Obere Bachstrasse 30 a, 94315 Straubing, Germany*

There are several disadvantages to fusion, such as obliteration of normal anatomy, elimination of movement, and increased stiffness. These disadvantages may increase the potential for other long-term complications ("fusion diseases") such as facet hypertrophy, facet arthritis, spinal stenosis, osteophyte formation, posterior muscular debilitation, and adjacent-level disc degeneration [1–6]. Motion-preserving techniques offer the opportunity to achieve intersegmental stabilization coupled with retained intersegmental mobility. Disc arthroplasty techniques may decrease transmission of detrimental stresses to the adjacent segments, which theoretically may counteract the early, accelerated degeneration often seen in these segments. Under proper adherence to their indications, these new motion-preserving techniques may help to avoid these fusion diseases.

Because the spinal motion segment consists of three well-balanced moving parts (ie, the intervertebral disc, the paired zygoapophyseal joints, and the surrounding soft tissue ligaments and muscles), some advanced-stage morphologic changes cannot be treated in an adequate manner with an anterior column disc replacement alone.

Types of hybrid constructs

Single-level hybrid constructs

Single-stage motion-preserving hybrid

Treatment with motion-preserving technologies should take into consideration all three moving parts of the motion segment. Thus, disc replacement technologies (nucleus replacement, total disc replacement) can be combined with posterior stabilizing elements (eg, dynamic pedicle screw–based devices, interspinous devices, or facet replacement) (Table 1, type 1).

Multistage motion-preserving hybrid

In this type of hybrid (see Table 1, types 2a and 2b), patients who already have an existing motion-preserving technology can have an additional one added later. This fact allows primary anterior and primary posterior technologies to be combined with secondary posterior or secondary anterior technologies in the future.

Multilevel hybrid constructs

Anterior motion-preserving technologies (nucleus replacement, total disc replacement) can be combined with posterior motion-preserving technologies (pedicle screw–based systems, interspinous devices, facet

---

* Corresponding author.
E-mail address: bertagnoli@pro-spine.com (R. Bertagnoli).

Table 1
Single-level hybrid constructs

Type	Level	Timing of surgical procedures	Type and location	
			Anterior	Posterior
1	Single	Single stage	yes	yes
2a	Single	Multistage	Previous surgery	yes
2b	Single	Multistage	yes	Previous surgery

replacement) at more than one level. The goal is to achieve three-dimensional, motion-preserving, biomechanically stable reconstruction of the involved motion segments, with a physiologic range of motion. Considering the treatment of a whole motion section, hybrids can be classified as follows:

Motion-preserving technologies combined with motion-preserving technology of any type (single-stage)

In this type of hybrid construct, only motion-preserving technologies are used (Table 2, type 3). Anterior technologies (nucleus replacement, total disc replacement) and posterior technologies (pedicle screw–based systems, interspinous devices, facet replacement) may be applied to different segments and combined in single segments. The goal of this kind of multilevel hybrid is to dynamically treat all of the affected spinal segments with motion-preserving technologies.

Motion-preserving technologies combined with fusion (single-stage)

If varying pathologies are found within multiple motion segments (eg, one segment has severe spondyloarthritis and complete segmental collapse, another segment has disc height reduced by 50%, and a third segment has a large central disc herniation—all without significant posterior element pathology), it makes no sense to reconstruct only the most affected motion segment with arthroplasty. In these cases, the application of a fusion technique in the lower or middle area can be considered so that a mechanically stable construct can be attained. This surgery is preferably done single stage (see Table 2, type 4).

Table 2
Multilevel hybrid constructs

Type	Level	Timing of surgical procedures	Type of procedure	
			Level x to z	Level y to z
3	multi	single stage	Motion-preservation techniques (anterior, posterior, or combinations)	Motion-preservation techniques (anterior, posterior, or combinations)
4	multi	single stage	Fusion procedure (any kind)	Motion-preservation techniques (anterior or posterior or combinations)
5a	multi	multistage	Previous surgery: fusion procedure (any kind)	Motion-preservation techniques (anterior, posterior, combinations)
5b	multi	multistage	Previous surgery: motion preservation (any kind)	Fusion procedure (any kind)

Motion-preserving technologies combined with previous fusion (multistage)

In the broadest sense, a hybrid is a combination of an already existing fusion with a motion-preserving technology (see Table 2, types 5a and 5b). This treatment is usually necessary due to a symptomatic adjacent-level instability. In these cases, the hybrids are created in different, consecutive surgical sessions. Anterior and posterior technologies or combinations of single-level hybrids can be applied.

Indications and contraindications to hybrid constructs

Indications

Because there is limited experience in combining these new technologies, indications for hybrid constructs are similar to those of the individual anterior motion-preserving devices (nucleus replacement, total disc replacement) or posterior dynamic devices

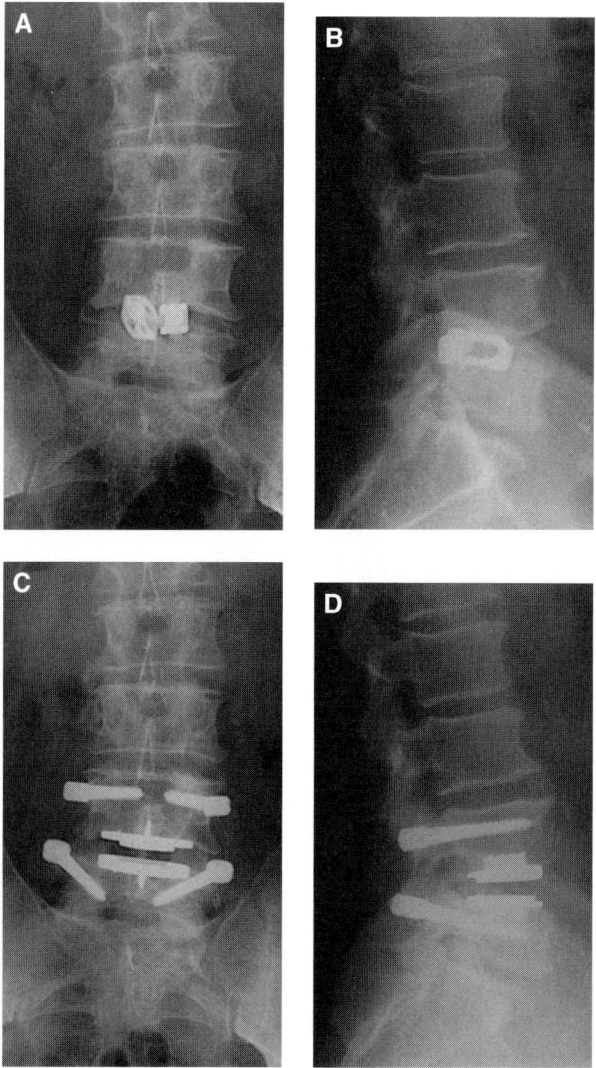

Fig. 1. Anteroposterior (*A*) and lateral (*B*) preoperative radiographs. Anteroposterior (*C*) and lateral (*D*) postoperative radiographs.

(pedicle screw–based systems, interspinous devices, facet replacement). Biomechanical and morphologic changes have to be taken into consideration to plan the reconstruction of a motion segment on a three-dimensional basis, which means the degree of degeneration and the degree of mechanical insufficiency must be considered by the surgeon before deciding on which technologies to combine.

Typical situations in which patients may benefit from hybrid constructs are multilevel-diseased spines in which all involved levels are symptomatic. These situations include multilevel degenerative disc disease with or without degenerative spondylolisthesis, degenerative scoliosis, combinations of isthmic or hypoplastic spondylolisthesis with degenerative disc disease–affected adjacent levels, breakdown of motion segments after fusion procedures, and many more situations that up to now have not been considered as candidates for a motion-preserving procedure.

Contraindications

The same contraindications that are considered for individual fusion and nonfusion technologies remain valid for these types of constructs. One of the biggest problems in considering motion preservation is osteoporosis or other major underlying bony pathologies (osteopenia, metastatic, or infectious diseases) that inherently reduce load-bearing capacities of the vertebral bodies and end plates. This is less of a concern in fusion-only reconstruction. In these conditions, the load-sharing capacities of any device that is anchored by pedicle screws or other fixation systems (posterior dynamic pedicle screw systems or interspinous systems) to the bony elements of the vertebrae or that rely on load transmission from one vertebral body to the other must be carefully considered preoperatively by the surgeon. Acute spinal fractures, spine tumors, discitis, and ventral approach–related problems are also generally considered contraindications [2]. In any surgical procedure, proper adherence to accepted indications is vital to achieve maximally successful postoperative results. As a good general rule, all conservative treatment options should be exhausted before surgery is undertaken.

Case studies

Hybrid construct type 1: Dynesys system plus ProDisc prosthesis

A 68-year-old man who had a previous fusion surgery at the L4-5 level using a posterior lumbar interbody fusion with two titanium-block cages de-

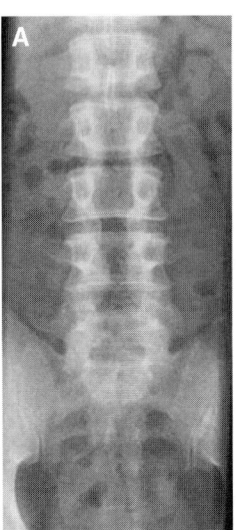
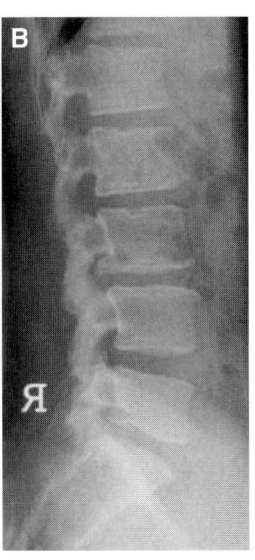
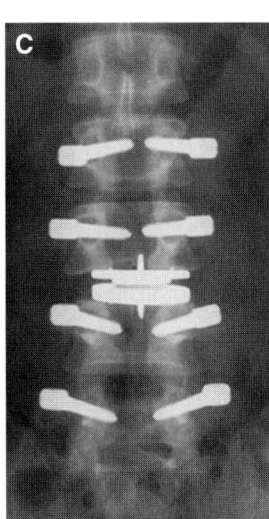
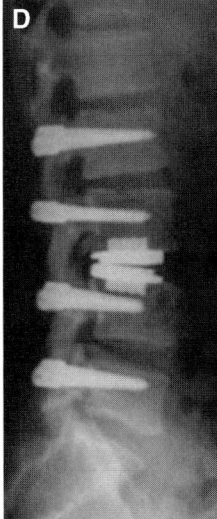

Fig. 2. Anteroposterior (*A*) and lateral (*B*) preoperative radiographs. Anteroposterior (*C*) and lateral (*D*) postoperative radiographs.

veloped persistent low back pain due to failure of bony incorporation through the implanted cages. In addition, later disc degeneration at the L3-4 and L5-S1 levels was diagnosed (Fig. 1A, B). In an anterior revision surgery, the cages were explanted and a ProDisc lumbar prosthesis (Synthes, Oberdorf, Switzerland) was implanted at the L4-5 level. In addition, a posterior reconstruction with dynamic instrumentation (the Dynesys system [Zimmer Spine, Warsaw, Indiana]) was performed at L4-5 as part of the same surgery. Postoperative radiographs showed good positioning of the implants (Fig. 1C, D). Within the first few days after surgery, a significant pain reduction was observed.

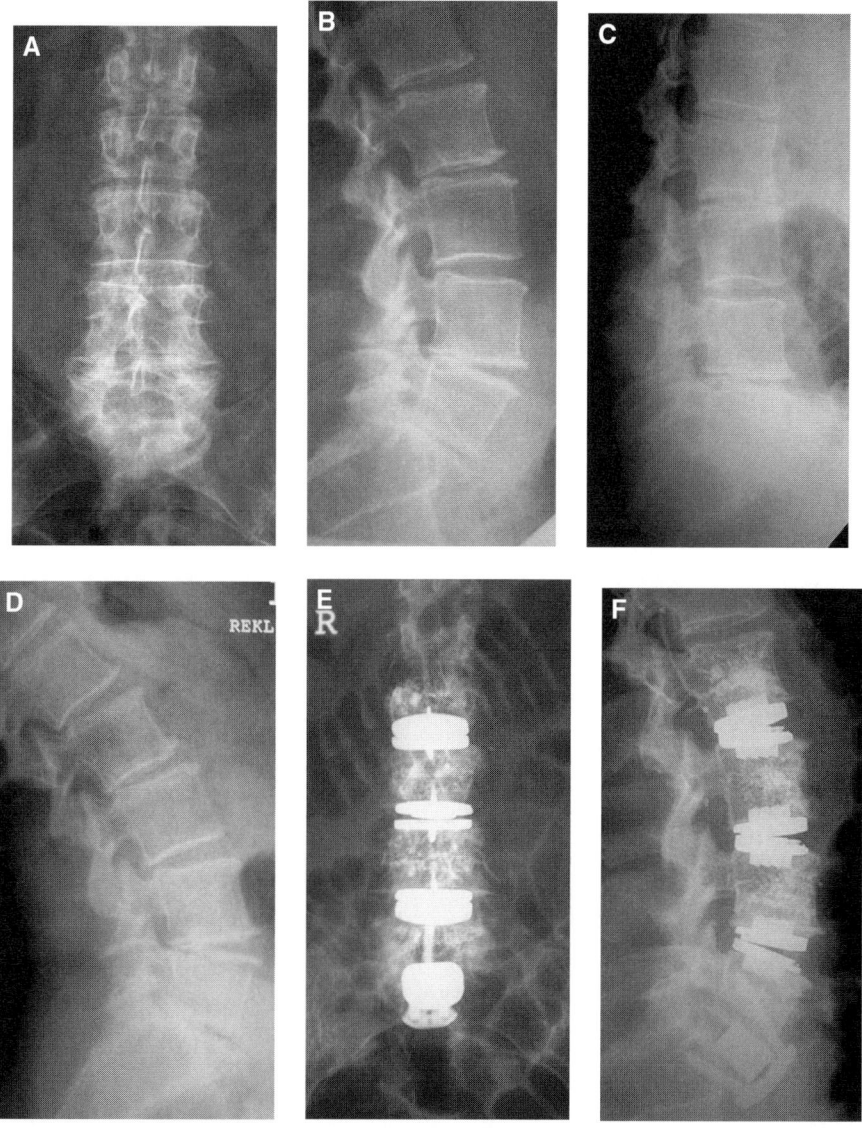

Fig. 3. Anteroposterior (*A*), lateral (*B*), flexion (*C*), and extension (*D*) preoperative radiographs. Anteroposterior (*E*), flexion (*F*), and extension (*G*) postoperative radiographs.

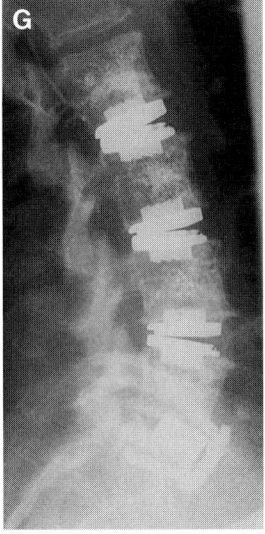

Fig. 3 (continued).

ment. He was several years postlaminectomy/discectomy at the L3-4 level and had developed degenerative disc disease at adjacent levels (Fig. 2A, B). The patient was treated with implantation of a ProDisc at the L3-4 level and dynamic instrumentation with the Dynesys system from L2 to L5 (Fig. 2C, D).

Hybrid construct type 4: anterior lumbar interbody fusion plus ProDisc (three-level)

A 61-year-old woman with disabling low back pain had a history of previous disc surgery at L4-5 and partial decompressive hemilaminectomies at L4-5 and L5-S1 (Fig. 3A–D). The recommended treatment was fusion surgery (anterior lumbar interbody fusion) at L5-S1 and multilevel arthroplasty surgery at the L2-3, L3-4, and L5-S1 levels with implantation of three ProDisc lumbar prostheses. In addition, vertebroplasty was performed at the L2 to L5 levels (Fig. 3E–G).

Hybrid construct type 3: ProDisc plus Dynesys system (three-level)

A 42-year-old man with a multiyear history of low back pain remained resistant to conservative treat-

Hybrid construct type 4: 360° fusion plus Pyramid plate plus ProDisc prosthesis

A 38-year-old female heavy manual worker with no previous surgery suffered from severe episodic

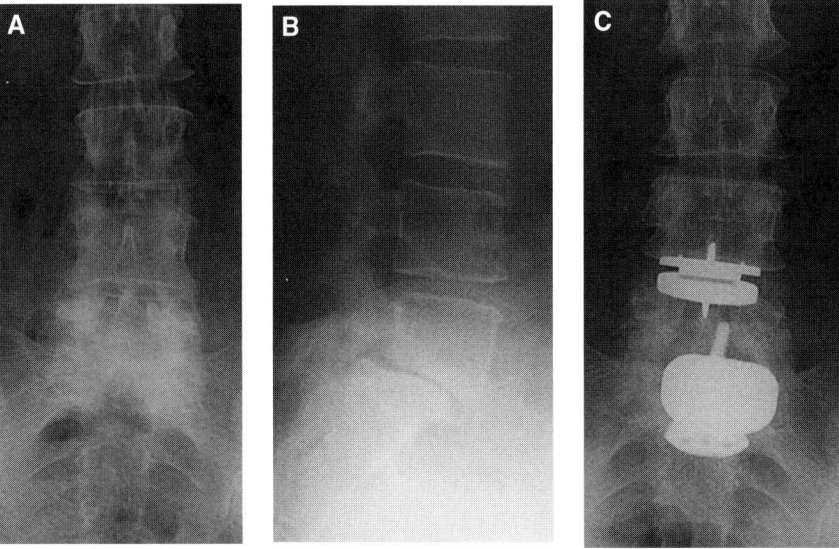

Fig. 4. Anteroposterior (*A*) and lateral (*B*) preoperative radiographs. Anteroposterior (*C*) and lateral (*D*) postoperative radiographs.

360° fusion using a ventral Pyramid plate (Medtronic Sofamor Danek, Memphis, Tennessee) and to implant a ProDisc prosthesis at the L4-5 level (Fig. 4C, D). At 1-year follow-up, the patient was completely satisfied with the surgery. The visual analog scale score declined from 8.0 preoperatively to 2.0 1 year postoperatively.

Hybrid construct type 4: anterior lumbar interbody fusion plus Maverick prostheses (two-level)

A 50-year-old woman suffered from low back pain for several years despite an attempted fusion at L3-4 (segment still unstable). Symptomatic degenerative disc disease at the L2-3 and L4-5 was also diagnosed. Surgical treatment was total disc replacement with Maverick prostheses (Medtronic Sofamor Danek, Memphis, Tennessee) at the L2-3 and L3-4 levels and an anterior lumbar interbody fusion at the L4-5 level. Postoperative radiographs showed correct positioning of the devices and a good restoration of disc height (Fig. 5A, B).

Hybrid construct type 5a: 360° fusion plus ProDisc prostheses (two-level)

A 38-year-old man had an L5-S1 360° fusion for disabling disc disease. He did well for 18 months

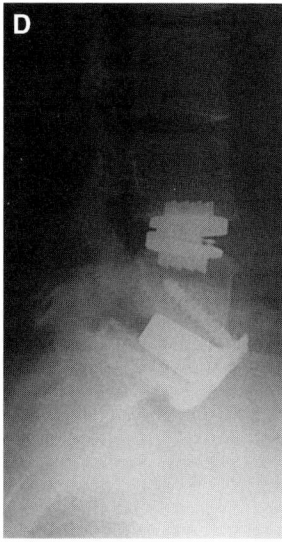

Fig. 4. (*continued*).

left leg pain and numbness in both legs. All nonsurgical treatment had failed. Radiographs demonstrated a grade I spondylolisthesis at the L5-S1 level and degenerative disc disease at L4-5 (Fig. 4A, B). It was elected to treat the L5-S1 level with a

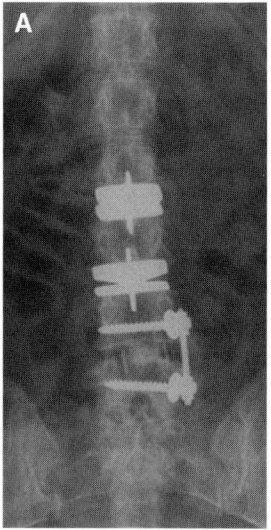
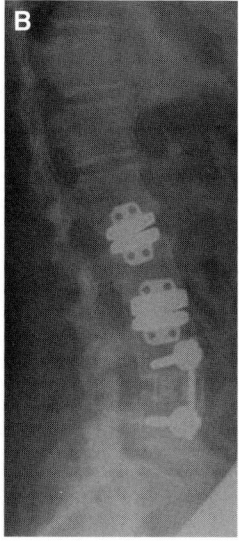

Fig. 5. Anteroposterior (*A*) and lateral (*B*) postoperative radiographs.

but developed progressively increasing pain. A new discogram at that time demonstrated internal disruption of L3-4 and L4-5, with significant pain reproduction at both levels. L2-3 was anatomically normal and painless. A special Compassionate Use waiver was obtained from the Food and Drug Administration to allow implantation of two ProDisc prostheses above his previous fusion (Fig. 6A–C). At 1-year follow-up, the patient is doing exceptionally well, working without restrictions, and delighted with his result.

Hybrid construct type 5a: posterior lumbar interbody fusion plus ProDisc prosthesis

A 45-year-old woman had a previous fusion surgery with posterior lumbar interbody fusion at the L5-S1 level in 1993. Eight years later, lumbar and radicular pain recurred (visual analog scale score: 8.0). Radiographs showed solid fusion at L5-S1 and instability at the L3-4 and L4-5 levels (Fig. 7A–C). All conservative treatment had failed. The patient was treated with implantation of a ProDisc lumbar pros-

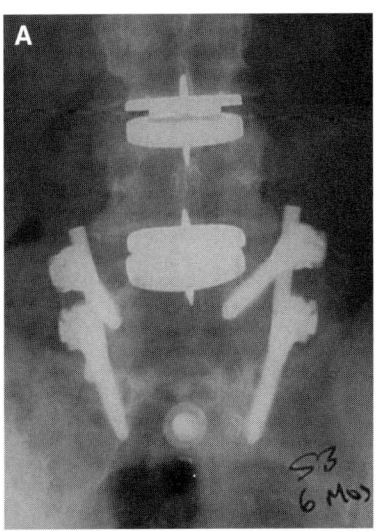
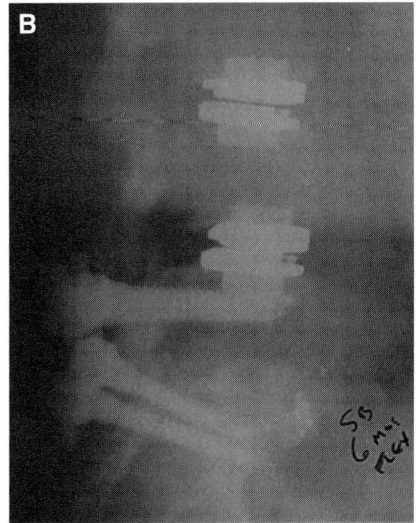
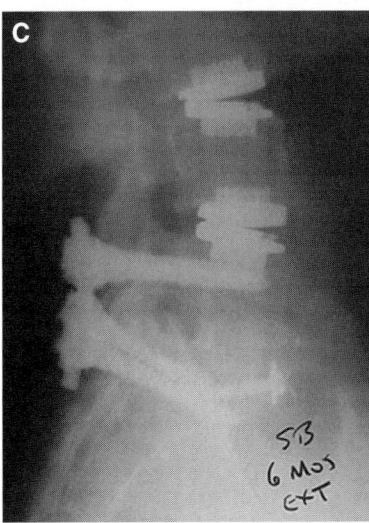

Fig. 6. Anteroposterior (*A*), flexion (*B*), and extension (*C*) postoperative radiographs.

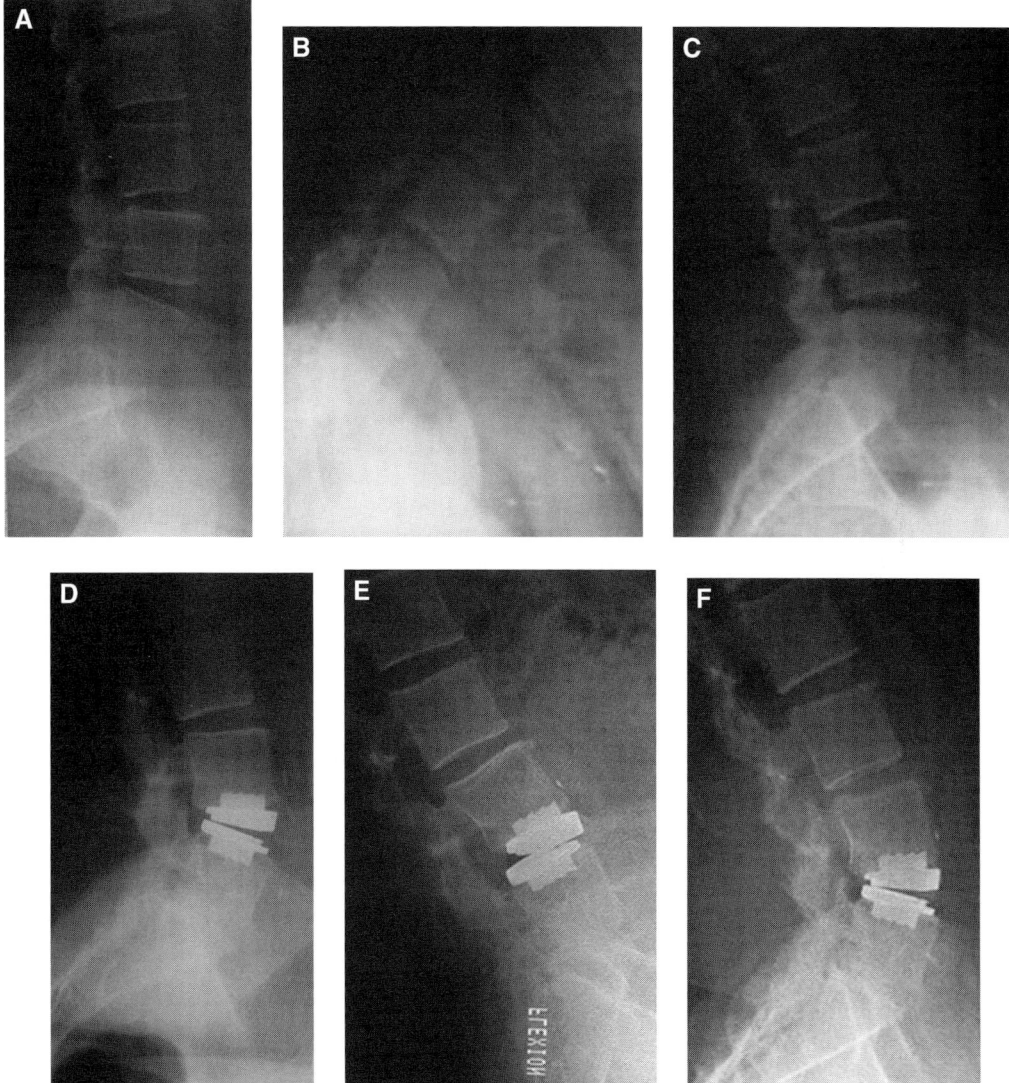

Fig. 7. Lateral (*A*), flexion (*B*), and extension (*C*) preoperative radiographs. Lateral (*D*), flexion (*E*), and extension (*F*) postoperative radiographs.

thesis only at the L4-5 level to re-establish lumbosacral lordosis. Postoperative radiographs showed good mobility of the prosthesis (Fig. 7D–F). Two years after surgery, the visual analog scale score was 2.0.

Summary

Because the spine is a very complex motion-serving organ consisting of three mobile columns, it may not be an ideal treatment strategy to replace only one of those columns. When the biomechanical insufficiency of all three columns is far advanced (eg, disc collapse following discectomy and posterior laminectomy or facetectomy), reconstruction of the posterior or anterior columns alone may result in an insufficient mechanical restoration of the motion segments, with persisting pain and disability. The mechanical necessity to control mobility in all three columns is more important in motion-preserving techniques than in fusion alone.

The promising results of anterior or posterior nonfusion techniques in single-column dysfunction have suggested an expansion of the indications in degeneratively diseased patients with multicolumn or multilevel pathologies. The authors' early experience with the limited expansion of current indications using a combination of motion-preserving technologies demonstrates promising results. Nevertheless, an expansion of these indications should only be performed under scientific scrutiny of those individuals in whom these techniques have been combined. This scientific scrutiny is particularly important because few of these technologies have prospective, nonrandomized data available for their isolated use, and the combination of these techniques in more complex situations increases the likelihood of complications. Short-, intermediate-, and long-term side effects of these combination therapies are currently unknown, and these patients must therefore be carefully followed so that the surgeon community can learn from these experiences. The casual use of these hybrid constructs should strictly be avoided. Furthermore, controlled single- and multicenter studies should be performed to explore the clinical value of the hybrid constructs described herein.

References

[1] Bertagnoli R. Disc surgery in motion. SpineLine 2004; 6:23–8.

[2] Bertagnoli R, Kumar S. Indications for full prosthetic disc arthroplasty: a correlation of clinical outcome against a variety of indications. Eur Spine J 2002; 11(Suppl 2):S131–6.

[3] Hilibrand AS, Robbins M. Adjacent segment degeneration and adjacent segment disease: the consequences of spinal fusion? Spine J 2004;4(Suppl 6):190S–4S.

[4] Malter AD, McNeney B, Loeser JD, et al. 5-year reoperation rates after different types of lumbar spine surgery. Spine 1998;23(7):814–20.

[5] Bono CM, Lee CK. The influence of subdiagnosis on radiographic and clinical outcomes after lumbar fusion for degenerative disc disorders: an analysis of the literature from two decades. Spine 2005;30(2):227–34.

[6] Bertagnoli R. Review of modern treatment options for degenerative disc disease. In: Kaech DL, Jinkins JR, editors. Spinal restabilization procedures. Diagnostic and therapeutic aspects of intervertebral fusion cages, artificial discs and mobile implants. Amsterdam: Elsevier; 2002. p. 365–75.

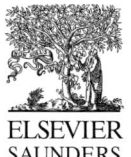

Complications and Strategies for Revision Surgery in Total Disc Replacement

Rudolf Bertagnoli, MD[a],*, Jack Zigler, MD[b], Armin Karg, MSc[c], Sandra Voigt, MSc[c]

[a]Spine Center, St.-Elisabeth-Klinikum, St.-Elisabeth-Str. 23, 94315 Straubing, Germany
[b]Texas Back Institute, 6300 West Parker Road, Plano, TX 75093-7916, USA
[c]Spine Center Straubing, Obere Bachstrasse 30 a, 94315 Straubing, Germany

As spinal arthroplasty becomes more widely available for the treatment of degenerative disc disease, it will likely replace fusion in many cases. To improve success using this motion-preserving treatment, accurate indications and precision in the implantation are required. In the European literature, the reported satisfaction rate for patient pain and function is up to 93% [1,2]. Although this new technology may offer benefits over arthrodesis, it requires the acquisition of new operative techniques and introduces a new spectrum of potential complications. Most of the complications in total disc replacement procedures are iatrogenic; wrong indications, poor implantation technique, and improper positioning of the implant are the most likely causes. Isolated device-related complications are rare (eg, subsidence, body fractures, polyethylene extrusion, and problems due to polyethylene wear). Due to stringently controlled inclusion groups, small study populations, and lack of long-term follow-up, only limited data are available. Lessons learned from hip and knee arthroplasty, however, suggest that the incidence of complications increases with duration of follow-up [3–5]. Recent reviews of spinal arthroplasty series have shown promising clinical outcomes with relatively low rates of reported complications [6–14], albeit in relatively short follow-up studies.

Complications

As in all procedures in which devices are implanted in the human body, complications can be separated into those related to the surgical approach, those related to implantation of the prosthesis, and those related to the interaction of the device with its host bed.

Approach-related complications

Currently available total disc replacement prostheses can be implanted only through an anterior approach. Therefore, approach-related complications are identical to those found in the anterior approach used in anterior lumbar fusion. Compared with wound infections, hematoma, and other lesser complications (like transient postoperative ileus), ureteral injuries, retrograde ejaculation, and great vessel injuries are the most significant and can lead to serious intraoperative complications. Among these complications, the great vessel injuries are the most serious and can be lethal if not immediately controlled.

Device-related complications

Device-related complications depend on the type of the device, the technique of insertion, and the primary and secondary fixation. In all of the different types of prostheses, subsidence is the most common problem. Most of the time, an inadequate

---

* Corresponding author.
E-mail address: bertagnoli@pro-spine.com (R. Bertagnoli).

determination of preoperative bone quality (introduction of an implant in a patient with osteopenia or osteoporosis) leads to subsidence of the prosthesis into the vertebral body. Subsidence has most frequently been reported within the first 3 months after implantation; late subsidence has rarely been reported.

Device migration or extrusion is mainly dependent on the primary and secondary fixation of the prosthesis. Implants with superior primary fixation (eg, prostheses with a keel) and prostheses incorporating a coating of the end plates allowing secondary osteointegration due to ongrowth or ingrowth to the surface of the prosthesis are superior to prostheses that do not have the ability for osteointegration. Other rare complications include splitting of the vertebral body following insertion of keeled implants or end plate or vertebral body fractures during the implantation.

Malposition of the prosthesis may result in foramenal narrowing, with dorsal root ganglion or nerve root compromise. Prostheses that require significant distraction during implantation of the device or polyethylene core may also lead to maintenance of an overdistraction. Root stretch can cause postoperative radicular pain of variable duration that may require treatment with medication, injections, or even spinal cord stimulation.

Normal movement within the implant produces wear. In devices in which a polyethylene core is used, polyethylene extrusion or polyethylene wear can eventually be seen. Metal-on-metal implants can potentially generate metal wear debris, which can be mechanically abrasive and biologically reactive.

Infection of the implant may also lead to a severe device-related complication potentially requiring revision anterior retroperitoneal or transperitoneal surgery, with increased morbidity.

More than 90% of device-related complications are iatrogenic. Poor patient selection, improper implantation, and wrong sizing are the most common examples of surgical errors causing a higher risk of failure.

Review of the literature shows that the incidence of device-related complications is low. Complication rates in different types of implants show an overall incidence of 1.5% to 4.0% [1–3].

Revision strategies

Patients with severe malposition, significant migration or extrusion, significant subsidence or body fractures, and infections of the device result in primary indications for revision surgery. In patients who have continued pain of unknown etiology, further evaluation of the pain source is necessary. If the implanted level is not the source, then additional levels may be responsible and an alternative treatment option such as creation of a hybrid construct may become necessary.

Wear debris can theoretically lead to a painful inflammatory response similar to that seen in total joint arthroplasty [15]. The long-term effects of wear debris in lumbar disc arthroplasty thus far remain unknown; however, existing literature reporting on long-term results (up to 20 years of follow-up in Europe) suggest a promisingly low incidence of wear-related problems in the spine.

Long-term mechanical failures of disc arthroplasty implants are unlikely, as suggested by mechanical testing [16]; compared with hip and knee joints, the overall mobility of discs is relatively low and the forces on the discs are not nearly as high.

Types of revision strategies

In principle, there are three main revision strategies. The first represents the case in which the anterior column prosthesis can be maintained if the mobility can be reduced or blocked. The range of mobility of the prosthesis can be reduced by inserting a posterior dynamic implant (pedicle screw–based or interspinous, resulting in a single-level hybrid) or eliminated using a fixed pedicle screw system and posterior lateral fusion or an anterior plate.

In the second revision strategy, the prosthesis (or some part of it) is replaced by a new one. In the third strategy, the prosthesis is completely removed from the anterior approach and replaced by an anterior interbody fusion.

The first strategy is the easiest and safest to implement because no revision anterior approach is necessary. Therefore, for cases in which the problems arise from the posterior elements such as facet arthrosis or hypermobility, posterior dynamic stabilization to unweight the posterior column and restrict segmental motion range may be an appropriate surgical solution. The second and third strategies are much more complicated because a revision anterior approach is required that carries with it a significantly higher approach-related complication rate. Because the great vessels have to be remobilized for revision spine surgery, an increased risk of intraoperative vascular injury with potentially severe consequences must be considered.

"Strategic" approach

A goal should be to keep the left-sided approach for the L4-5 region virgin for as long as possible because it is the most difficult level to reach. One strategy might be to recommend that index surgeries at the L5-S1 level be done from the right side so that a revision surgery, which might be necessary in the future at that level, can be done by a transperitoneal approach. This strategy also keeps the left-sided approach available for more proximal levels if they break down in the future.

Insertion of an antiadhesive membrane

Another strategy to make vascular dissection easier and safer is to use an anti-adhesive membrane (eg, Gore-Tex, W. L. Gore & Associates, Inc., Newark, Delaware). This membrane is inserted between the prosthesis and the great vessels during the primary surgery. In a revision surgery, the vessels can more easily be dissected from the anterior spine and mobilized to the right side Another way to reduce adhesions between the great vessels and the spine is to keep manipulation of the vessels to a minimum with gentle surgical technique, thus minimizing fibrosis between the vessels and the spine.

Prostheses with a modular design

Prostheses with a modular design in which the wearing part can be separately exchanged without disturbing the bone–implant interface are advantageous for revision surgery purposes because the entire prosthesis does not have to be replaced. This design limits the amount of vascular exposure needed and does not require bony resection. Implants that can be inserted through a lateral or oblique approach may have an easier and safer revision potential.

When the decision is made to explant the device and fuse the segment, the revision intervention should ideally be performed from an oblique or lateral approach to avoid significant manipulation of the great vessels, which is especially critical in the L4-5 area. By performing oblique or lateral partial corpectomy, even prostheses with a fixation keel can be removed without significant vascular manipulation.

Cases

Various types of complications with different prostheses

- Charité (Johnson & Johnson De Puy Acromed, Raynham, Massachusetts): subsidence (Fig. 1).
- ProDisc (Synthes, Oberdorf, Switzerland): subsidence 4 days post surgery into posterior part of end plate L5 due to osteoporosis (wrong indication) (Fig. 2).
- Maverick (Medtronic Sofamor Danek, Memphis, Tennessee): body splitting (Fig. 3).

Case studies

Explantation of ProDisc with subsequent anterior fusion (complication occurred due to trauma)

A 39-year-old woman had been treated with implantation of a ProDisc prosthesis at the L5-S1 level. Three months after surgery, the patient fell on her buttocks, causing an impaction fracture of the upper end plate of the prostheses into the L5 vertebral body (Fig. 4A, B). Conservative treatment for 3 more months could not reduce the level of her persistent increased low back pain. Six months after implantation, revision surgery with implant removal and anterior cage and plate fixation was performed (Fig. 4C, D). After this surgery, her low back pain was completely resolved.

Vertebral body fracture

A 53-year-old woman underwent an uncomplicated two-level ProDisc implantation (Fig. 5A, B). She was osteopenic, with a preoperative T score of

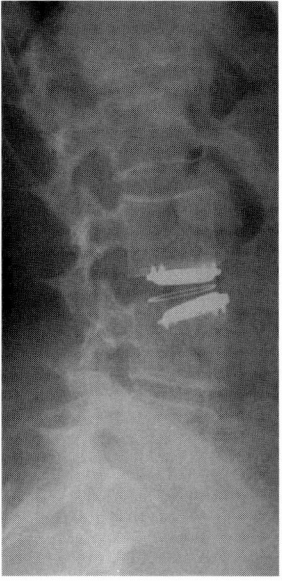

Fig. 1. Lateral postoperative radiograph showing subsidence of Charité prosthesis.

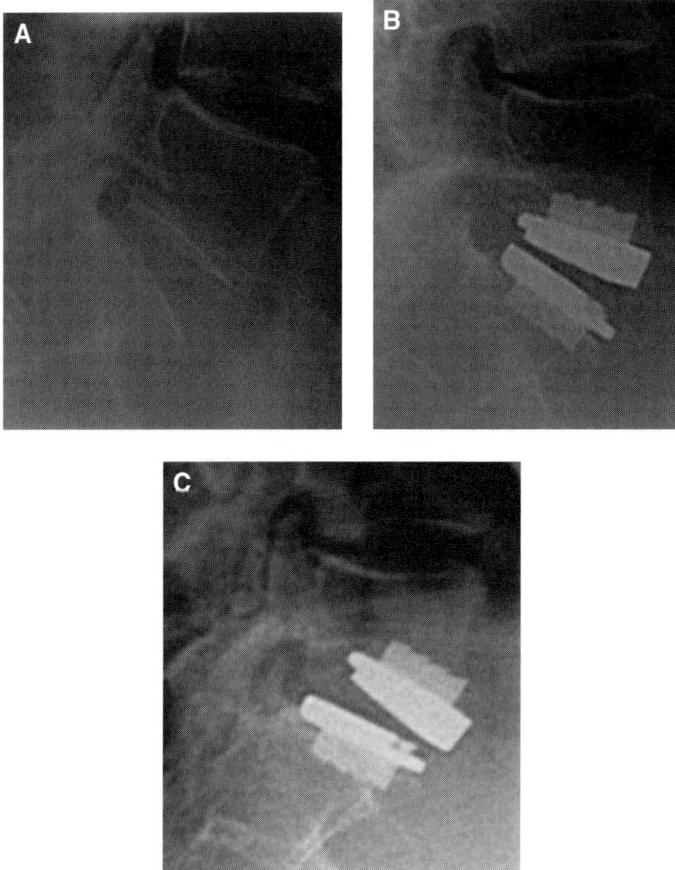

Fig. 2. (*A*) Lateral preoperative radiograph. (*B*) One-day postoperative radiograph. (*C*) Four-day postoperative radiograph showing subsidence.

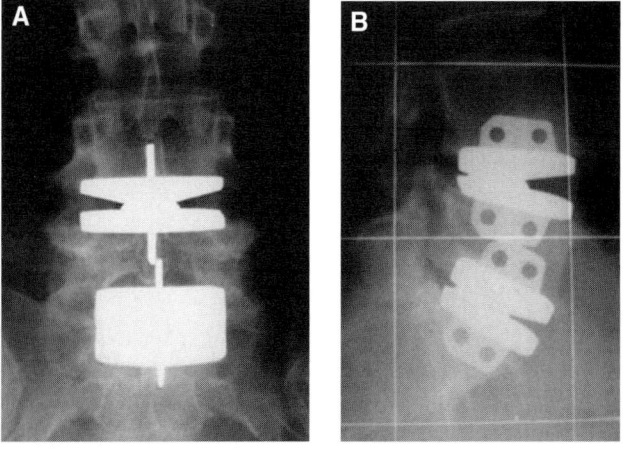

Fig. 3. Anteroposterior (*A*) and lateral (*B*) postoperative radiographs.

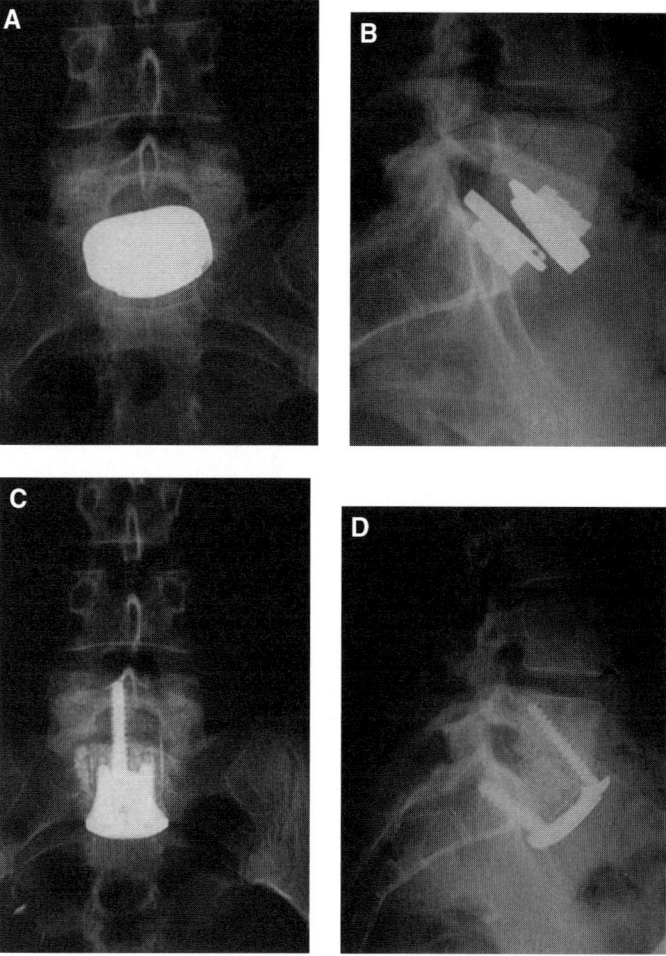

Fig. 4. Anteroposterior (*A*) and lateral (*B*) postoperative radiographs showing subsidence. Anteroposterior (*C*) and lateral (*D*) postoperative radiographs after revision surgery with anterior fusion plus pyramid plate system.

−2.3. After surgery, she was constipated and treated with medication. Six days postoperatively, while straining at stool, she experienced sudden severe pain in her back with tingling in her left leg. Emergency radiographs showed an L5 vertebral body fracture (Fig. 5C). Revision surgery with removal of both implants and L5 vertebrectomy with anterior reconstruction and posterior instrumented fusion was performed (Fig. 5D, E). The patient improved after surgery and was able to return to work as a nurse 4 months post surgery. Some persistent low back pain was maintained.

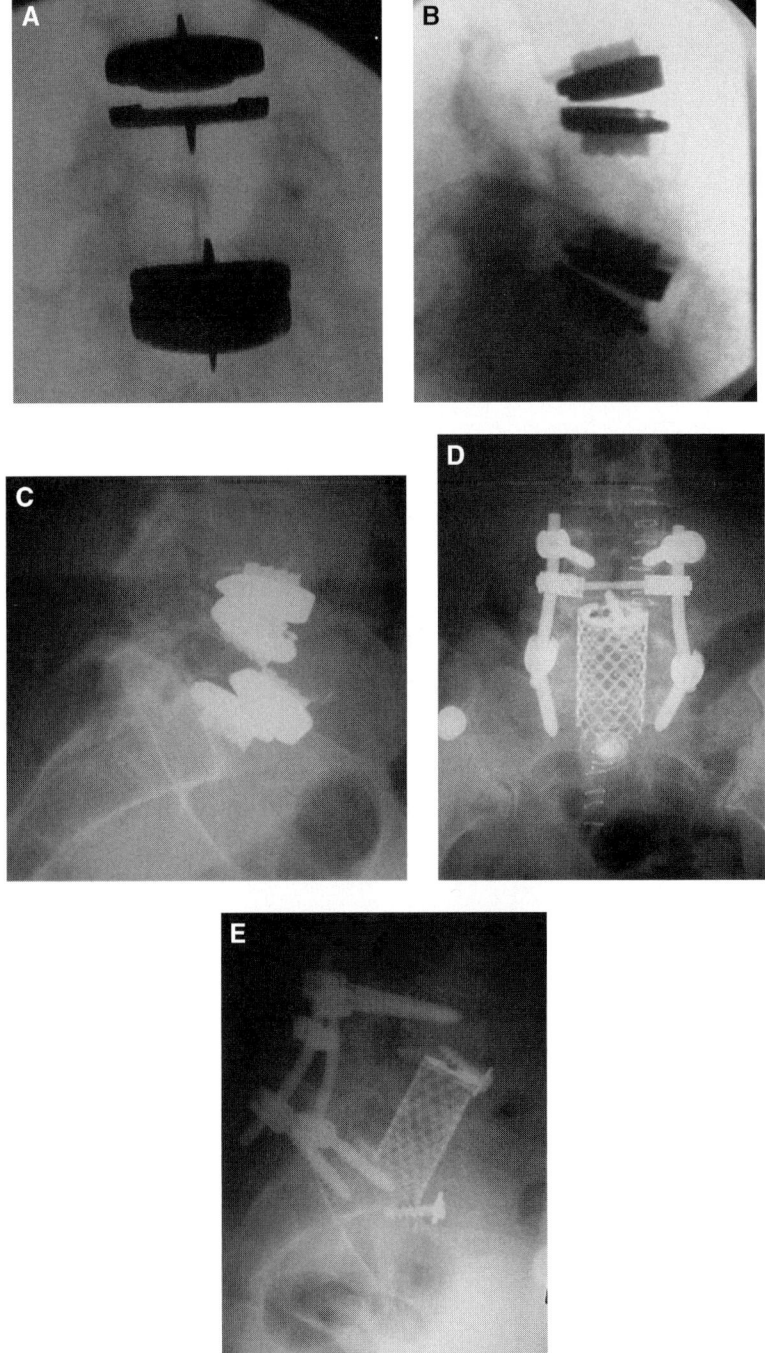

Fig. 5. Anteroposterior (*A*) and lateral (*B*) intraoperative radiographs. (*C*) Lateral postoperative radiograph showing L5 vertebral body fracture. Anteroposterior (*D*) and lateral (*E*) postoperative radiographs after revision surgery with anterior and posterior fusion.

Summary

Even though total disc replacement in the cervical and lumbar spine appears to be a relatively safe and efficacious surgical option for degenerative disc disease (as evidenced by patient follow-up data) and has low overall complication rates not dissimilar to anterior fusion surgery, the potential for complications and salvage must be considered. To avoid complications, systematized preoperative diagnostic and patient selection processes are very important. Of crucial importance are sizing, positioning, and anticipated kinematics of the implant. Appropriate surgeon training regarding implantation techniques, good fluoroscopic control during implantation, and expertise in the anterior approach are essential. Salvage procedures for failed total disc arthroplasty can most easily consist of posterior/lateral fusion, simple addition of a posterior dynamic stabilization device, or a posterior instrumented fusion when the implant can be left as an anterior column strut. A more difficult option is an anterior revision approach with component replacement or complete device removal and anterior fusion. Due to the high vascular risk in anterior revision surgeries, these latter options should be performed only in specialized spine centers with a large experience in anterior approaches, using an experienced vascular surgical team. A revision anterior approach should primarily be considered only when the implant must be removed for anterior migration causing vascular compromise or infection.

References

[1] Bertagnoli R, Yue J. The treatment of disabling single level lumbar discogenic low back pain with total disc arthroplasty utilizing the PRODISC prosthesis: a prospective study with 2 year minimum follow-up. Spine J (accepted).

[2] Bertagnoli R, Yue J. The treatment of disabling multilevel lumbar discogenic low back pain with total disc arthroplasty utilizing the Prodisc prosthesis: a prospective study with 2 year minimum follow-up. Spine J (accepted).

[3] van Ooij A, Oner FC, Verbout AJ. Complications of artificial disc replacement: a report of 27 patients with the SB Charité© disc. J Spinal Disord Tech 2003;16: 369–83.

[4] Griffith SL, Shelokov AP, Buttner-Janz K, et al. A multicenter retrospective study of the clinical results of the LINK SB Charite intervertebral prosthesis. The initial European experience. Spine 1994;19:1842–9.

[5] Lemaire JP, Skalli W, Lavaste F, et al. Intervertebral disc prosthesis. Results and prospects for the year 2000. Clin Orthop 1997;337:64–76.

[6] Anderson PA, Rouleau JP, Toth JM, et al. A comparison of simulator-tested and -retrieved cervical disc prostheses. Invited submission from the Joint Section Meeting on Disorders of the Spine and Peripheral Nerves, March 2004. J Neurosurg Spine 2004;1(2): 202–10.

[7] Anderson PA, Sasso RC, Rouleau JP, et al. The Bryan Cervical Disc: wear properties and early clinical results. Spine J 2004;4:S303–9.

[8] Goffin J, Casey A, Kehr P, et al. Preliminary clinical experience with the Bryan Cervical Disc Prosthesis. Neurosurgery 2002;51:840–5.

[9] Goffin J, Van Calenbergh V, van Loon J, et al. Intermediate follow-up after treatment of degenerative disc disease with the Bryan Cervical Disc Prosthesis: single-level and bi-level. Spine 2003;28:2673–8.

[10] Duggal N, Pickett GE, Mitsis DK, et al. Early clinical and biomechanical results following cervical arthroplasty. Neurosurg Focus 2004;17:62–8.

[11] McAfee PC, Cunningham B, Dmitriev A, et al. Cervical disc replacement-porous coated motion prosthesis: a comparative biomechanical analysis showing the key role of the posterior longitudinal ligament. Spine 2003;28:S176–85.

[12] Pimenta L, McAfee PC, Cappuccino A, et al. Clinical experience with the new artificial cervical PCM (Cervitech) disc. Spine J 2004;4:S315–21.

[13] Traynelis VC. The Prestige cervical disc replacement. Spine J 2004;4:S310–4.

[14] Robertson J, Porchet F, Brotchi J, et al. A multicenter trial of an artificial cervical joint for primary disc surgery. Presented at the Society for Spinal Arthroplasty. Montpellier, France, May 2002.

[15] Hallab NJ, Cunningham BW, Jacobs JJ. Spinal implant debris-induced osteolysis. Spine 2003;28:S125–38.

[16] Kostuik JP. Complications and surgical revision for failed disc arthroplasty. Spine 2004;4:289–91.

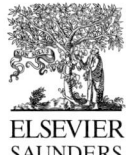

Index

Note: Page numbers of article titles are in **boldface** type.

A

Adjacent level degeneration
   reduction of, 264–265

Anterior lumbar interbody fusion plus Maverick prostheses, 385

Anterior lumbar interbody fusion plus ProDisc prosthesis, 384

Arthropathy
   lumbar disc
      contraindications to, 296
      indications for, 296

B

Bone graft
   need for
      elimination of, 263–264

Bristol Disc
   for cervical total disc replacement, 360–362
      evolution of, 360–361
      improved clinical trials, 361–362
      pilot study, 361
      refined designs, 361–362

Bryan Cervical Disc prosthesis
   for cervical total disc replacement, 358–360
      complications with, 360
      design of, 358
      results with, 358–360

C

Cervical spine
   anatomy of, 349–350
   degenerative disorders of, **255–262.** See also *Degenerative disorders, of lumbar and cervical spine.*
      described, 259–260
      treatment of, 260–261
   pathophysiology of, 349–350

Cervical total disc replacement, **349–354**
   biomaterials in, 351
   biomechanics in, 351
   clinical results of, **355–362**
      Bristol Disc, 360–362
      Bryan Cervical Disc prosthesis, 358–360
      ProDisc-C, 355–358
   implant types in, 352–353
      metal-on-metal designs, 352
      metal-polymer designs, 352–353
   indications for, 350–351
   rationale for, 350

Charité lumbar total disc replacement, 296–297
   clinical results of, 332–334
   complications of, 334–340
   contraindications to, 325–326
   described, 323
   immediate postoperative period, 331
   indications for, 324–325
   operative technique, 328–331
   patient positioning for, 328
   preoperative planning for, 326–328
   prosthetic implantation in, 328–331
   rehabilitation after, 331–332
   spine biomechanics and, 323–324
   surgical approach to, 328

D

Degenerative disc disease
   pathophysiology of, 294
   prosthetic nucleus for, 342
   treatment of
      nonsurgical, 294–295
      surgical, 295

Degenerative disorders
   of lumbar and cervical spine, **255–262.** See also *Cervical spine, degenerative disorders of; Lumbar spine, degenerative disorders of.*
      degenerative process in, 256–257
         disc composition and structural effects in, 256–257

nutritional changes in, 257
vascular changes in, 257
pain generation in, 257–258
treatment of, 260–261

Disc(s)
intervertebral. See *Intervertebral disc.*

Dynamic Stabilization System for the Spine (DYNESYS), **363–372**
clinical results with, 368–370
concept of, 364–365
described, 363–364
indications for, 366–368
philosophy of, 364–365

DYNESYS. See *Dynamic Stabilization System for the Spine (DYNESYS).*

Dynesys system plus ProDisc prosthesis, 382–383

F

Flexicore
in lumbar total disc replacement, 297

G

Graf ligamentoplasty, **373–377**
biomechanics of, 373–374
clinical results of, 375–376
described, 373
indications for, 374–375

H

Hybrid constructs, **379–388**
case studies, 382–387
contraindications to, 382
indications to, 381–382
multilevel, 379–381
multistage motion-preserving hybrid, 379
single-level, 379
types of, 379–381
type 1, 382–383
type 3, 384
type 4, 384–385
type 5a, 385–387

I

Implant(s). See specific types, e.g., *Nuclear implants.*

Intervertebral disc
anatomy of, 255–256, 293–294
biomechanics of, 294
degenerative process of, 256–257
normal, 255–256
physiology of, 255–256, 293–294

L

Ligamentoplasty
Graf, **373–377**. See also *Graf ligamentoplasty.*

Lumbar disc arthropathy
contraindications to, 296
indications for, 296

Lumbar partial disc replacement, **341–347**
disc mechanics and physiology in, 341–342
indications for, 344–345
nucleus replacement devices in
development of, 342–343
types of, 343–344
results of, 345–346

Lumbar spine
degenerative disorders of, **255–262**. See also *Degenerative disorders, of lumbar and cervical spine.*
described, 258
treatment of, 260–261
lower
anterior miniopen retroperitoneal approach to, 286–287
standard and minimally invasive approaches to
posterior approach, 287–291
Wiltse approach, 288

Lumbar total disc replacement, **293–299**
contraindications to, 296
history of, 295
ideal characteristics of, 295
implants for
types and characteristics of, 296–297
indications for, 296
Maverick
clinical results of
two-year prospective follow-up, **315–322**. See also *Maverick lumbar total disc replacement, clinical results of, two-year prospective follow-up.*
postoperative care, 298
ProDisc-II
clinical results of, **301–313**. See also *ProDisc-II lumbar total disc replacement.*
SB Charité, 296–297, **323–340**. See also *Charité lumbar total disc replacement.*
surgical considerations in, 297–298

M

Maverick lumbar total disc replacement, 297
 clinical results of
  two-year prospective follow-up, **315–322**
   complications of, 318–319
   discussion of, 320–321
   materials and methods in, 315–318
   radiologic results of, 319–320
   results of, 318–320

Multilevel hybrid constructs, 379–351

Multistage motion-preserving hybrid, 379

N

Nonfusion implants
 advantages of, 263–265
 biomechanics of, **271–280**
 disadvantages of, 265–267

Nonfusion technology
 in spine surgery
  advantages and disadvantages in, **263–269**. See also *Spine surgery, nonfusion technology in.*

Nuclear implants
 biomechanics of, 276

Nucleus(i)
 prosthetic
  for degenerative disc disease, 342

Nucleus replacement devices
 for lumbar partial disc replacement
  development of, 342–343
  types of, 343–344

P

Pain
 in degenerative disorders of lumbar and cervical spine, 257–258
  motion segment–related, 257
  neural compression–related, 257–258

Posterior lumbar interbody fusion plus ProDisc prosthesis, 386–387

Posterior stabilization devices
 biomechanics of, 276–277

ProDisc
 in lumbar total disc replacement, 296

ProDisc implant, 301–303

ProDisc plus Dynesys system, 384

ProDisc-C
 for cervical total disc replacement, 355–358
  design of, 355
  indications for, 355
  results with, 357–358
  surgical approach for, 356–357

ProDisc-II lumbar total disc replacement
 clinical results of, **301–313**
  case studies, 310–313
  discussion of, 309–310
  U.S. pivotal clinical trial, 302–309
   design of, 303
   estimated motion from flexion-extension radiographs in, 308–309
   outcome instruments, 304–305
   outcome measures, 307–308
   radiographs in, 305
   results of, 307
   statistical analysis, 305–307
   surgical technique, 303–304
 ProDisc implant for, 301–303

Prosthesis(es)
 anterior lumbar interbody fusion plus Maverick, 385
 anterior lumbar interbody fusion plus ProDisc, 384
 Bryan Cervical Disc, 358–360. See also *Bryan Cervical Disc prosthesis.*
 Dynesys system plus ProDisc, 382–383
 implantation of
  in Charité lumbar total disc replacement, 328–331
 posterior lumbar interbody fusion plus ProDisc, 386–387
 360-degree fusion plus ProDisc, 385–386
 360-degree fusion plus Pyramid plate plus ProDisc, 384–385

Prosthetic nucleus
 for degenerative disc disease, 342

Pseudoarthrosis
 elimination of, 264

R

Radiography
 of ProDisc-II lumbar total disc replacement, 305

Rehabilitation
 after Charité lumbar total disc replacement, 331–332

Revision surgery
 in total disc replacement, **389–395**. See also *Total disc replacement, revision surgery in.*

S

SB Charité
  in lumbar total disc replacement, 296–297
    clinical results of, **323–340.** See also *Charité lumbar total disc replacement.*

Segment(s)
  fused
    biomechanics of, 273

Single-level hybrid constructs, 379

Spinal loading
  anatomy and, 271–272

Spinal unit
  functional
    diseased, 272–273
    normal, 271–272

Spine
  cervical. See *Cervical spine.*
    standard and minimally invasive approaches to, 282–285
      anterior approach, 284–285
      posterior approach, 282–284
        anatomy related to, 282
        incision and dissection in, 282
        minimally invasive, 282–284
        positioning in, 282
  lumbar. See *Lumbar spine.*
    standard and minimally invasive approaches to, **281–292**
      anterior thoracolumbar extensile approach, 285–286
      anterolateral transpsoatic approach, 287
      complications of, 291
      thoracic approach to, 285–291
      thoracolumbar approach, 285–291

Spine surgery
  nonfusion technology in
    advantages and disadvantages in, **263–269**
    nonfusion implants
      advantages of, 263–265
      disadvantages of, 265–267

T

360-degree fusion plus ProDisc prostheses, 385–386

360-degree fusion plus Pyramid plate plus ProDisc prosthesis, 384–385

Total disc replacement
  biomechanics of, 273–276
  cervical, **349–354.** See also *Cervical total disc replacement.*
  lumbar, **293–299.** See *Lumbar total disc replacement.*
  revision surgery in, **389–395**
    complications of, 389–390
      approach-related, 389
      case studies, 391–394
      device-related, 389–390
      strategies for, 390–391

NO POSTAGE
NECESSARY
IF MAILED
IN THE
UNITED STATES

BUSINESS REPLY MAIL
FIRST-CLASS MAIL   PERMIT NO 7135   ORLANDO FL

POSTAGE WILL BE PAID BY ADDRESSEE

PERIODICALS ORDER FULFILLMENT DEPT
ELSEVIER
6277 SEA HARBOR DR
ORLANDO FL 32821-9816